Clinical
Calculations

APPROXIMATE EQUIVALENTS

1 gr = 60 mg

15 gr = 1 Gm = 1000 mg

1000 mcg (μg) = 1 mg

1 kg = 2.2 lb

1 ml (1 cc) = 15 m

4 ml (4 cc) = 1 dr (ℨ)

5 ml (5 cc) = 1 tsp (t)

30 ml (30 cc) = 1 oz (℥) = 2 tbsp (T) = 6 tsp (t) = 8 dr (ℨ)

500 ml (500 cc) = 1 pt (0) = 16 oz (℥)

1000 ml (1000 cc) = 1 L = 1 qt = 32 oz (℥)

Clinical Calculations

A Unified Approach

THIRD EDITION

Joanne M. Daniels, RN, BSN, MSN
Professor Emeritus
SUNY College of Technology at Alfred, Alfred, NY

Loretta M. Smith, RN, BSN, MEd.
Professor Emeritus
SUNY College of Technology at Alfred, Alfred, NY

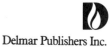
Delmar Publishers Inc.

I(T)P™

NOTICE TO THE READER

Cover:
   Ed Atkeson, Berg Design

Delmar staff:
   Administrative Editor: Patricia Casey
   Project Editor: Melissa Conan
   Production Coordinator: Mary Ellen Black
   Art and Design Coordinator: Mary Siener

For information, address Delmar Publishers Inc., 3 Columbia Circle, Box 15015, Albany, NY 12203-5015

Printed in the United States of America
Published simultaneously in Canada by Nelson Canada,
a division of The Thomson Corporation

   3 4 5 6 7 8 9 10   XXX   00 99 98 97 96 95 94

Library of Congress Cataloging-in-Publication Data
Daniels, Joanne M.
   Clinical calculations : a unified approach / Joanne M. Daniels,
Loretta M. Smith.—3rd ed.
      p.   cm.
   Includes index.
   ISBN 0-8273-5945-4
   1. Pharmaceutical arithmetic.   2. Drugs—dosage.   3. Drugs—
Administration.   4. Nursing—Mathematics.   I. Smith, Loretta M.
II. Title.
   [DNLM: 1. Drugs—administration & dosage—nurses' instruction.
2. Mathematics—nurses' instruction.   3. Weights and Measures—
nurses' instruction.   QV 16 D186c 1994]
RS57.D36   1994
615'.14—dc20
DNLM/DLC
for Library of Congress   93-19225
                                                               CIP

Contents

....

Preface   xi
    Acknowledgments   xiii

Unit I   **The Label Factor Method**   1
    Introduction   1
    Overview: The Label Factor Method   2
    Relationships and Rationale   4
    Accuracy and Accountability   16

Unit II   **The Metric System of Measurement**   17
    Basic Units   17
    Metric Abbreviations   17
    Metric Notation   17
    Comparing Metric Units   17
    Converting Units Within the Metric System   19

Unit III   **The Apothecaries System of Measurement**   24
    Basic Units and Abbreviations   24
    Apothecaries Notation   25
    Comparing Apothecaries Units   26
    Converting Units Within the Apothecaries System   26

Unit IV   **The Household System of Measurement**   30
    Household Units   30
    Household Notation   31
    Comparing Household Units   31
    Converting Units Within the Household System   32

Unit V   **Conversion of Metric, Apothecaries, and Household Units**   35
    Self-Quiz—Equivalents   35
    Conversion from One System to Another   38

Unit VI   **Calculation of Oral Medications**   45
    Oral Medications   45
    The Medicine Cup   46
    Rounding Off   47
    Reading Labels and Calculating Dosage   49
    Calculations Based on Body Weight   57

Unit VII   **Administration of Oral Medications**   71
    Medication Order   71
    Abbreviations   73

	Self-Quiz—Abbreviations	75
	Routes for Administering Medications	76
	The Medication Kardex (Medex)	76
	Recording Medications	78
	Drug Distribution System	78
	Accountability	79
	General Rules for Administration of Medications	79
	Administering Oral Medications	80
	Performance Criteria: Administration of Oral Medications	82
Unit VIII	**Calculation of Parenteral Medications**	**90**
	Parenteral Medications	90
	The Syringe and Needle	91
	Reading the Syringe	93
	Rounding Off	95
	Parenteral Medication Forms	97
	Reading Labels	99
	Calculating Dosages Obtained from Pre-mixed Solutions	105
	Calculations Based on Body Weight	115
	Units of Medication	118
	Reconstitution of Drugs in Powder Form	122
Unit IX	**Administration of Parenteral Medications**	**132**
	Injection Sites and Techniques	132
	Precautions in Handling Needles and Syringes	138
	Administration of Parenteral Medications	140
	Performance Criteria: Administration of Injections	141
	Variation of Parenteral Injection Techniques: IM	147
	Performance Criteria: Z-Track Method—Deep Intramuscular Injection	147
	Variation of Parenteral Injection Techniques: SC	149
	Performance Criteria: Administration of Heparin	149
	Insulin Preparations	151
	Insulin Administration	157
	Performance Criteria: Administration of Insulin	160
Unit X	**Calculations of Intravenous Medications and Solutions**	**162**
	Intravenous Injections and Infusions	162
	Equipment	163
	Reading Labels: Drop Factor	166
	Reading IV Labels	168
	Intermittent IV Drug Administration	170
	Intravenous Regulators	173
	Calculation of Intravenous Flow Rates, Infusion Times, Infusion Rate, and Bolus Using Label Factor Method	176

Calculation of IV Flow Rate When Total Infusion Time Is Specified — 177

Calculation of IV Flow Rate When an Infusion Rate Is Specified — 177

Calculation of Flow Rate (GTT/MIN) When IV Contains Medication — 182

Calculation of IV Flow Rate When an Infusion Pump is Used — 183

Calculation of Infusion Time — 186

Adding Medications to Intravenous Fluids — 188

Adding Drugs to IVs and Calculating the Drug Infusion Rate — 196

Calculating IV Dosage and Flow Rate Based on Body Weight — 204

Titrated Infusions — 210

Drugs Administered by IV Bolus — 219

Parenteral Nutrition — 224

Assessment and Adjustment — 228

Unit XI   Administration of Intravenous Medications and Solutions   235

Intravenous Administration — 235

Infusion Sites — 236

Nursing Responsibilities Relative to Intravenous Administration — 236

Precautions in Handling IV Equipment — 238

Recording — 239

Performance Criteria: Setting Up an IV — 239

Performance Criteria: Starting IV — 241

Performance Criteria: Assessment, Adjustment, and Termination of IV — 243

Unit XII   Pediatric Dosage   245

General Considerations in Administering Oral and Parenteral Medications to Children — 245

Administration of Parenteral Medications to Infants and Children — 246

Pediatric Dosage Based on Body Weight—Oral Medications — 248

Calculating Pediatric Dosage—Injections — 254

Calculating Pediatric Dosage—IVs — 257

Calculation of Pediatric Dosage Based on Body Surface Area — 263

Application of Label Factor Method Using BSA Estimates — 265

Unit XIII   Clinical Calculations   267

Appendix A Arithmetic Review   325

Appendix B Percentage Solutions   343

Appendix C Answer Keys   349

Index   371

Index of Tables

Table 1-1 Conversion Equation   7
Table 1-2 Approximate Equivalents   7
Table 1-3 Sequential Conversion Factors   8
Table 2-1 Metric Units   18
Table 2-2 Metric Prefixes   18
Table 2-3 Metric Abbreviations   18
Table 2-4 Metric Notation   18
Table 2-5 Metric Units of Weight   19
Table 2-6 Metric Units of Volume   19
Table 2-7 Metric Units of Length   19
Table 3-1 Basic Apothecaries Units   25
Table 3-2 Apothecaries Notation   25
Table 3-3 Apothecaries Fluid Units   27
Table 4-1 Household Units   31
Table 4-2 Household Equivalents   31
Table 4-3 Household Notation   32
Table 5-1 Approximate Equivalents Among Metric,
           Apothecaries, and Household Systems   36
Table 7-1 Amount/Dosage   73
Table 7-2 Preparations   73
Table 7-3 Routes   74
Table 7-4 Times   74
Table 7-5 Special Instructions   75
Table 10-1 Conversion Between ml/hr and gtt/min   185

Preface

● ●

CLINICAL CALCULATIONS offers students and practitioners alike the opportunity to develop skill in solving dosage problems using the label factor method (also known as dimensional analysis). This method is a logical and systematic approach to solving any type of medication administration problem. The method can be used with any system of measurement and facilitates conversion from one system to another. It easily replaces all other procedures for calculating medication dosages.

The advantages of a unified approach to clinical calculations include protection and precision, as well as ease and efficiency. The variety of approaches to dosage computations can be confusing and perplexing. A logical system is needed to reduce significantly errors made when medications are administered or dispensed. The label factor method is such a system.

The text applies this versatile method to a cross section of computational applications typical of the clinical setting. These applications include calculating adult and pediatric oral and parenteral dosages, as well as intravenous flow rates and infusion times. Numerous solved examples guide the learner in using the method for these applications. Self-quizzes provide the opportunity for learners to practice the label factor method. The text also includes a detailed review of the routes by which medications are administered, particularly as they relate to the different types of dosage calculations. Performance criteria checklists for each route of administration provide a means of documenting learner progress in mastering the techniques.

This textbook is suitable for use in either traditional lecture classes, small group tutorial classes, or self-instruction. The third edition contributes to the self-instructional mode of learning. It provides more detailed explanations of the label factor method as it is used in different applications to help learners understand the method. More than 100 new drug labels familiarize learners with commonly prescribed drugs and provide opportunities for hands-on computation practice. All drugs have been updated and identified by generic names. New content includes use of label factor method for nutritional calculations and titration of infusions. In addition, the arithmetic review section has been amplified with respect to multiplying and dividing fractions and decimals.

Content

Unit 1 introduces the label factor method, teaches the basic steps, and provides practice problems for each step as well as for the entire procedure.

Units 2–5 review the three systems of measurement (metric, apothecaries, and household) commonly used in prescribing medications and apply the label factor method to conversions within and between the systems.

Units 6 and 7 focus on medications administered by the oral route. The label factor method is used in Unit 6 to determine dosages of medications, both liquid and solid. In Unit 7, general considerations related to safe and effective administration of oral medications and performance criteria are included, as are terms and abbreviations.

Units 8 and 9 apply the label factor method to dosage computations for medications administered parenterally (exclusive of intravenous administration), specifically via intradermal, subcutaneous, and intramuscular routes. General considerations, methodology, equipment, location of sites, and performance criteria are included in Unit 9.

Units 10 and 11 focus on intravenous computations and administration. In Unit 10 the label factor method is applied to the various computational problems associated with intravenous (IV) flow rate, infusion times, titrated medication additives, infusions, and parenteral nutrition. Unit 11 describes the various routes of IV administration and includes sample problems related to each route.

Unit 12 applies the label factor method to the calculation of pediatric dosages based on body weight or body surface area. Also included are general considerations related to administering medications to infants and children.

Unit 13 summarizes the application of the label factor method. Two hundred twenty clinical problems offer a variety of examples of all of the preceding types of calculations. This unit can serve as a performance evaluation tool and a useful reference or review.

The Appendix section of the text contains three parts. Although it is assumed that learners using this text are familiar with elementary mathematics, Appendix A includes a variety of drill problems for review or practice in basic arithmetic processes. Students who require additional review or remediation are encouraged to seek the assistance of faculty or other sources.

Appendix B applies the label factor method to the calculation of components for the preparation of percentage solutions.

Finally, Appendix C contains the answers to all of the self-quizzes and problems in the text.

A useful adjunct to the text for teachers looking for additional problems is an Instructor's Guide containing the answers to all quizzes and solutions to all practice problems, and a test bank covering Units 6–13 of the text with problem solutions.

Acknowledgments

We wish to express our sincere appreciation to the many individuals whose interest and assistance sustained and supported our efforts throughout the revision of this text.

We are especially grateful to our colleagues and reviewers for their constructive and instructive critiques as well as their excellent ideas and suggestions, which have added new depth and dimension to the present edition. Their advocacy and encouragement, along with that of our families and friends, were invaluable and inspiring, and helped to make this endeavor an exciting and rewarding experience.

Appreciation is expressed also to the following agencies and companies that supplied labels and photographs for illustrations and permission for use of copyrighted materials:

Abbott Laboratories, Abbott Park, IL
A. H. Robins Company, Richmond, VA
Armour Pharmaceutical Company, Fort Washington, PA
Arrow International, Inc., Reading, PA
Bard Med Systems Division, North Reading, PA
Baxter Healthcare Corporation, Deerfield, IL
Beecham Laboratories, Bristol, TN
Boehringer Ingelheim Pharmaceuticals, Inc., Ridgefield, CT
Bristol-Myers Company, Evansville, IN
Burroughs Wellcome, Research Triangle Park, NC
Eli Lilly and Company, Indianapolis, IN
Elkins-Sinn, Inc., Cherry Hill, NJ
G. D. Searle and Company, Chicago, IL
Hoechst-Roussel Pharmaceuticals Inc., Somerville, NJ
IVAC Corporation, San Diego, CA
Janssen Pharmaceutical, Inc., Piscataway, NJ
John C. Moore Corporation, Rochester, NY
Lederle Laboratories, Pearl River, NY
Lypho Med, Inc., Rosemont, IL
Marion Laboratories, Inc., Kansas City, MO
McNeil Pharmaceutical, SpringHouse, PA
Mead Johnson, Evansville, IN
Merrell Dow Pharmaceuticals, Inc., Cincinnati, OH
Pfizer Laboratories Division, New York, NY
Quad Pharmaceuticals, Inc., Indianapolis, IN
Roerig Pfizer, New York, NY
Roxane Laboratories, Inc, Columbus, OH

Smith Kline & French Laboratories, Philadelphia, PA
Squibb-Novo, Inc., Princeton, NJ
W. B. Saunders Company, Philadelphia, PA
Winthrop Laboratories, New York, NY
Wyeth-Ayerst, New York, NY
Wyeth Laboratories, Philadelphia, PA

Last, but surely not least, our loving thanks to Stu and Ang for fealty, fortitude, and forebearance above and beyond the call of husbandry.

The following individuals who reviewed the complete manuscript provided valuable guidance to the authors in preparing the final text. Their contributions are gratefully acknowledged.

Louann Boose
Harrisburg Area Community
  College
Shermansdale, PA

Marilyn Martis
Lorain County Community
  College
N. Royalton, OH

Patricia Reustle, RN, MS
Vocational Nursing Department
San Jacinto College
Houston, TX

Connie Houser, RNG, MSN
Central Carolina Technical College,
  formerly Sumter Area Technical
  College
Sumter, SC

The Label Factor Method

•••

Objectives

Upon completion of this unit of study you should be able to:
- *Analyze computation problems in order to identify the starting factor and the label for the answer.*
- *Analyze computation problems to identify equivalents given and equivalents needed.*
- *Set up an appropriate sequence of labeled factors, called a conversion equation, whereby successive labels can be cancelled.*
- *Correctly solve the conversion equation using cancellation and arithmetic to arrive at the desired labeled answer.*

This text presents a comprehensive approach to clinical calculations which is unique, uniform, and understandable. The term *clinical calculations* refers to the solving of computational problems associated with the administration of medications, specifically, determining the correct dosage to be given. Because these computations often involve converting from one system of measurement to another, it is essential that an accurate, reliable, and consistent method of solving conversion problems be utilized.

Introduction

Many drug and dose calculation textbooks dealing with mathematics relative to clinical practice use the methods of *ratio and proportion* and/ or *desire over have times quantity* for the conversion of units of measure. Where two or more conversions are involved, these methods often become cumbersome and confusing to the learner. Frequently, the learner must "remember" a certain procedure or a different approach for each type of problem. This attempt to memorize several procedures involving similar units may be perplexing and discouraging.

We attempt to bring order out of confusion by using a consistent method, the *label factor method,* for all conversion problems.

This method focuses on the particular labeled quantity in a problem for which an answer is sought and which is called the *starting factor.* With consistent practice, the learner soon develops the ability to find this key item. From this point on, emphasis is placed on a cancellation process whereby equivalent values, called *conversion factors,* are converted from one system of units to another, leading, finally, to the desired answer. These conversion factors fall into two categories. They are relationships that either (a) have been learned or (b) are obtainable from tables. The continuous emphasis on these relationships and their labeled units means that they become very familiar and recognizable to the learner and, soon, this familiarity facilitates almost automatic application of the method to all conversion problems. Once the technique has been mastered, all other formulas or methodologies can be discarded.

Other advantages of the label factor method include:

- The learner develops the ability to analyze all problems in a systematic manner.
- Memorization of different procedures for various types of problems is eliminated.
- The simplest arrangement of terms is obtained to facilitate cancellation and combination.
- Common mistakes of reverse operations (multiplying instead of dividing) are minimized.
- A continuous dimensional analysis of units is used to obtain a *properly labeled result.*
- The systematic approach develops an ability to solve new problems as they occur in the field.
- Many students are already familiar with the label factor method, because it is a computational technique taught in basic chemistry courses. Application of the method to clinical calculation is both rapid and facile.

Overview: The Label Factor Method

Definitions:

1. The *label factor method,* also known as *dimensional analysis,* is a computation method whereby one particular unit of measurement is converted to another unit of measurement by use of a conversion factor or factors.
2. A *conversion factor* is an equivalent value that can be used as a bridge between units of measurement without changing their value.

Steps in the Label Factor Method

The label factor method consists of three steps:
1. Determining the starting factor and answer label.
2. Formulating a conversion equation consisting of a sequence of labeled factors, in which successive labels can be cancelled until the desired answer label is reached.
3. Solving the conversion equation by use of cancellation and simple arithmetic.

Application of the Label Factor Method

Problem: How many seconds are there in 5 minutes?

Step I—Determining the Starting Factor and Answer Label

To solve this problem, it is necessary to convert from minutes to seconds. Therefore, the starting factor should be minutes and the answer label should be seconds. When the computation has been completed, these two units of measurement will have an equivalent relationship.

Example: 5 min = _____ sec

Step II—Formulating the Conversion Equation

An equivalent value that can be used as a bridge from minutes to seconds is:

$$60 \text{ sec} = 1 \text{ min}$$

Note that this is a 1 : 1 relationship (i.e., conversion factor), which can be written:

$$\frac{60 \text{ sec}}{1 \text{ min}} \text{ or } \frac{1 \text{ min}}{60 \text{ sec}}$$

The conversion equation is formulated so it will cancel all labels except the designated answer label.

Example: $5 \text{ \cancel{min}} \times \dfrac{60 \text{ sec}}{1 \text{ \cancel{min}}} = $ _____ sec

Step III—Solving the Conversion Equation

Cancellation of labels, reduction of numerical values, and simple multiplication are used to solve the conversion equation.

Example: $5 \text{ min} \times \dfrac{60 \text{ sec}}{1 \text{ min}} = 300 \text{ sec}$

Note that the starting factor, 5 min, and the labeled answer, 300 sec, have now formed an equivalent relationship; that is, 5 minutes has been converted to 300 seconds. Thus, the label factor method has been applied to convert one particular unit of measurement to another unit of measurement without changing the values.

Relationships and Rationale

The foregoing is a condensed overview of the label factor method. The following section offers analysis and amplification of the technique, plus practice and drill in its application. The content is subdivided into the three component steps of the label factor method.

Step I—Determining the Starting Factor and Answer Label

Initially, it is essential to determine exactly what information is sought. This information goal usually is indicated by a question or request to find something. For example:

Find the number of milliliters in 4 qts   Determine the number of cups in 4 qts
How many ounces are contained in 4 qts?   Calculate how many pints equal 4 qts

In each of these instances, an equivalent amount is sought for the quantity 4 quarts. Thus, 4 quarts is a particular *labeled value* that must be converted to an equivalent value to solve a problem or answer a question. In the label factor method, this labeled value, 4 quarts, is called—as we said—the starting factor. The label of the equivalent value to which the starting factor will be converted is called the *answer label*. In the earlier example, the answer labels are: milliliters, ounces, cups, and pints. With this in mind, what information is sought in the following questions:

1. How many 10 grain tablets are needed to administer 1 gram of a medication?
   Answer: 1 gram is the particular labeled value that must be converted to the equivalent value (number) of 10 grain tablets. The starting factor, therefore, is "1 gram" and the answer label is "tablets."

2. How many minims are contained in 1 teaspoon?
   Answer: 1 teaspoon is the labeled value that must be converted to the equivalent value (number) of minims. The starting factor, therefore, is "1 teaspoon" and the answer label is "minims."
3. What is the weight in kilograms of a child weighing 40 pounds?
   Answer: 40 pounds is the labeled value that must be converted to the equivalent value (number) of kilograms. The starting factor, therefore, is "40 pounds" and the answer label is "kilograms."

Some problems may contain a variety of information that may confuse the learner during identification of the starting factor and answer label. However, with careful reading and specific attention directed at the labeled value for which an equivalent value is sought, the learner soon develops proficiency in sorting out these two values.

Examples:

a. How many feet are there in 12 yards?
   Starting Factor   Answer Label
        12 yd   ft
b. How many inches are there in 29 feet?
   Starting Factor   Answer Label
        29 ft   in
c. How many ounces are there in 6 cups?
   Starting Factor   Answer Label
        6 cups   oz

Practice: Identifying the Starting Factor and Answer Label

1. How many milligrams are there in 3 grains?
   Starting Factor   Answer Label
   _____   _____

2. How many pounds are there in 5 kilograms?
   Starting Factor   Answer Label
   _____   _____

3. How many tablets should the patient receive if the physician ordered 250 milligrams?
   Starting Factor   Answer Label
   _____   _____

4. How many capsules should the patient receive if the ordered dose was 0.5 grams?
   Starting Factor   Answer Label
   _____   _____

5. How many milliliters should be administered if the dose is 250 milligrams?
   Starting Factor   Answer Label
   _____   _____

(*Note:* See Appendix C for answer key)

> **Remember:** The starting factor is always the first item in the label factor equation. The answer label is always the final item in the equation. When the label factor equation is solved, it will be seen that the starting factor and the labeled answer have formed an equivalent relationship.

Step II—Formulating the Conversion Equation

The second step in the label factor method is to set up a *sequential* series of *equivalent values* whereby successive labels can be cancelled until the only label remaining is the desired label for the answer. These equivalent values are called *conversion factors,* Table 1-1. It is essential that conversion factors contain only true $(1:1)$ relationships; that is, the numerator and denominator of each factor must be equivalent values. Because multiplying a number by 1 does not change the number, adding conversion factors to the equation does not change the value of the answer.

It is important to note that conversion factors may be constant or variable relationships. *Constant* relationships are absolutes; they do not vary regardless of the context in which they are used, Table 1-2. On the other hand, *variable* relationships, such as price, weight, and dosage, do not necessarily remain constant, as illustrated in the following examples.

Examples:

Constant Relationships	Variable Relationships
a. Equivalent Value: 15 gr = 1 Gm	a. Equivalent Value: 350 mg = 1 tab
Conversion Factor: $\dfrac{15\,\text{gr}}{1\,\text{Gm}}$ or $\dfrac{1\,\text{Gm}}{15\,\text{gr}}$	Conversion Factor: $\dfrac{350\,\text{mg}}{1\,\text{tab}}$ or $\dfrac{1\,\text{tab}}{350\,\text{mg}}$
b. Equivalent Value: 1 kg = 2.2 lb	b. Equivalent Value: 350 mg = 2.5 ml
Conversion Factor: $\dfrac{1\,\text{kg}}{2.2\,\text{lb}}$ or $\dfrac{2.2\,\text{lb}}{1\,\text{kg}}$	Conversion Factor: $\dfrac{350\,\text{mg}}{2.5\,\text{ml}}$ or $\dfrac{2.5\,\text{ml}}{350\,\text{mg}}$
c. Equivalent Value: 1 tsp = 5 ml	c. Equivalent Value: 350 mg = 1 tsp
Conversion Factor: $\dfrac{1\,\text{tsp}}{5\,\text{ml}}$ or $\dfrac{5\,\text{ml}}{1\,\text{tsp}}$	Conversion Factor: $\dfrac{350\,\text{mg}}{1\,\text{tsp}}$ or $\dfrac{1\,\text{tsp}}{350\,\text{mg}}$

Table 1-1. CONVERSION EQUATION

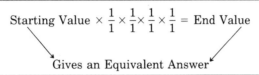

Table 1-2. APPROXIMATE EQUIVALENTS

$$1 \text{ gr} = 60 \text{ mg}$$
$$15 \text{ gr} = 1 \text{ Gm} = 1000 \text{ mg}$$
$$1000 \text{ mcg } (\mu\text{g}) = 1 \text{ mg}$$
$$1 \text{ kg} = 2.2 \text{ lb}$$
$$1 \text{ ml } (1 \text{ cc}) = 15 \text{ m}$$
$$4 \text{ ml } (4 \text{ cc}) = 1 \text{ dr } (\text{Ʒ})$$
$$5 \text{ ml } (5 \text{ cc}) = 1 \text{ tsp } (\text{t})$$
$$30 \text{ ml } (30 \text{ cc}) = 1 \text{ oz } (\text{Ʒ}) = 2 \text{ tbsp } (\text{T}) = 6 \text{ tsp } (\text{t}) = 8 \text{ dr } (\text{Ʒ})$$
$$500 \text{ ml } (500 \text{ cc}) = 1 \text{ pt } (0) = 16 \text{ oz } (\text{Ʒ})$$
$$1000 \text{ ml } (1000 \text{ cc}) = 1 \text{ L} = 1 \text{ qt} = 32 \text{ oz } (\text{Ʒ})$$

Approximate equivalents sometimes fall within a range, e.g., 60–65 mg = 1 gr, 4–5 ml = dr 1, 15–16 m = 1 ml. In addition, the pint and quart equivalents are rounded from 480 ml to 500 ml and 960 ml to 1000 ml, respectively. For purposes of clinical calculations in this text, the numbers in Table 5-1 will be used.

Key to Abbreviations:

gr = grain	gtt = drop	tbsp (T) = tablespoon
mg = milligram	ml = milliliter	pt (0) = pint
Gm = gram	cc = cubic centimeter	L = liter
kg = kilogram	dr (Ʒ) = dram	qt = quart
lb = pound	tsp (t) = teaspoon	
m, ℳ = minim	oz (Ʒ) = ounce	

Remember: It is essential that conversion factors be arranged so that similar labels are placed diagonally; that is, whatever label appears in the numerator of one factor appears in the denominator of the factor immediately following. For example:

$$1 \text{ cup} \times \frac{1 \text{ qt}}{4 \text{ cups}} \times \frac{1 \text{ gal}}{4 \text{ qt}}$$

Thus, it can be seen that labels can be logically and sequentially cancelled, greatly reducing the chance of error or omission. In solving the problem, each numerator cancels out the immediately following denominator, so that all labels are removed until the desired label for the answer is reached. For instance: the label (gal), which cannot be cancelled by a subsequent label, ends the equation and is the answer label that was identified in Step I.

> **Remember: Prior to setting up the sequence of labeled conversion factors, the starting factor and answer label must have been identified and these become, respectively, the first and last items in the equation, forming an equivalent relationship.**

Setting Up the Sequence of Conversion Factors   Study Table 1-3 to view the step-by-step sequence of conversion factors that lead from the starting factor to the answer. The problem requires changing a distance

Table 1-3.   SEQUENTIAL CONVERSION FACTORS

Problem: Change 500 yards to another distance.

Starting Factor	Conversion Factor(s)		Answer Label
a. 500 yd ×	$\frac{}{\text{yd}}$	=	_____ ?
b. Change 500 yd to inches			
500 yd ×	$\frac{36 \text{ in}}{1 \text{ yd}}$	=	_____ in
c. Change 500 yd to miles			
500 yd × $\frac{3 \text{ ft}}{1 \text{ yd}}$ ×	$\frac{1 \text{ mi}}{5,280 \text{ ft}}$		_____ mi

of 500 yards to something else. The purpose of the first conversion factor is to "cancel the label" in the starting factor, therefore the corresponding label is placed in the denominator as shown at (a). In (b), the answer is required in inches, therefore the factor converting yards to inches is used. If the answer is required in miles, two factors would be used as in (c), changing yards to feet and then to miles. Note that the conversion factors cease when the answer label is reached.

The learner may find it helpful to list the equivalent values that lead from the starting factor to the answer, prior to using them as conversion factors. The equivalent values in the problem below are: 1 yd = 36 in, 1 yd = 3 ft, and 5,280 ft = 1 mi. Study the following problem, which further illustrates the identification of equivalent values.

Problem 1: Find the number of yards in 1.5 miles.

  Equivalents: 1 mi = 5,280 ft; 3 ft = 1 yd

Now write the conversion equation:

Starting Factor	**Conversion Factors**	**Answer Label**
1.5 m̶i̶	$\times \quad \dfrac{5,280 \text{ f̶t̶}}{1 \text{ m̶i̶}} \times \dfrac{1 \text{ yd}}{3 \text{ f̶t̶}}$	$= \quad \underline{\hspace{2cm}}$ yd

The following observations regarding the above problem summarize Step II of the label factor method.

■ The starting factor is 1.5 mi, because this is the labeled value for which an answer (equivalent value) is sought.
■ In the two conversion factors, the labels *mile* and *feet* are placed in the denominators to cancel the corresponding labels of the immediately preceding factors. (*Note:* Make this a cardinal rule for the label factor method—that *each factor cancels a label in the preceding factor.*)
■ The two conversion factors, 5,280 ft/mi and 1 yd/3 ft, are each equivalent relationships. That is, these factors have 1 : 1 value and do not change the actual value of the starting factor. Their purpose is to lead to an equivalent answer expressed in some other unit. The relationship in *each* factor must be true for the answer to be correct.
■ The answer label always appears in the numerator farthest to the right in the conversion equation (in the example above: 1 yd).

Approximate Equivalents   In setting up conversion factors, the learner either must know the equivalent relationships in various systems of measurement or have this information available for reference. Because it is frequently necessary to convert from one system of measurement to another in the same problem, the use of exact equivalents for corresponding units often results in large and cumbersome fractions or decimals that are very inconvenient in calculations and that may contribute to error. Therefore, certain *approximations* have been accepted widely and are in general use as equivalents for converting between systems. Table 1-2 lists *approximate equivalents* that are most frequently used in the calculation of medication dosages or solutions.

Identifying Equivalents Using Table 1-2, list all the equivalents needed to solve the following problems, then set up the conversion equation.

Problem 1: How many 0.5 pint bottles can be filled by 4 quarts of solution?

Analysis of the question identifies 4 quarts as the starting factor and bottles as the answer label. Therefore, the equation involves going from 4 quarts to an equivalent number of bottles. The steps would include quarts to pints to bottles.

Equivalents: 1 qt = 2 pts, 1 bottle = 0.5 pt

Conversion Equation:

Starting Factor		**Conversion Factors**		**Answer Label**
4 quarts	$\times$	$\dfrac{2\,\text{pints}}{1\,\text{quart}} \times \dfrac{1\,\text{bottle}}{0.5\,\text{pint}}$	=	_____ bottles

Problem 2: Change 250 mg to Gm.

Equivalents: 1 Gm = 1000 mg

Conversion Equation:

Starting Factor		**Conversion Factors**		**Answer Label**
250 mg	$\times$	$\dfrac{1\,\text{Gm}}{1000\,\text{mg}}$	=	_____ Gm

---

Remember: In setting up the conversion factors, it is helpful to write the denominator first, as this will contain the label of the preceding numerator and facilitate cancellation of successive labels. Then, write the equivalent value in the numerator and proceed in this fashion for successive factors.

Problem 3: Find the number of minims in 3 teaspoons.

Equivalents: 1 tsp = 5 ml, 1 ml = 15 m

Conversion Equation: $3 \text{ tsp} \times \dfrac{5 \text{ ml}}{1 \text{ tsp}} \times \dfrac{15 \text{ m}}{1 \text{ ml}} = $ _____ m

Problem 4: 0.5 lb is equivalent to how many milligrams?

Equivalents: 2.2 lb = 1000 Gm, 1 Gm = 1000 mg

Conversion Equation: $0.5 \text{ lb} \times \dfrac{1000 \text{ Gm}}{2.2 \text{ lb}} \times \dfrac{1000 \text{ mg}}{1 \text{ Gm}} = $ _____ mg

Problem 5: Change 5 grains to grams.

Equivalents: 15 gr = 1 Gm

Conversion Equation: $5 \text{ gr} \times \dfrac{1 \text{ Gm}}{15 \text{ gr}} = $ _____ Gm

Note that the last equation shows the most direct route from grains to grams. However, it can be seen from Table 1-2 that other equivalent relationships exist between grains and grams.

Examples:

a. Equivalents: 15 gr = 1000 mg, 1000 mg = 1 Gm

Conversion Equation: $5 \text{ gr} \times \dfrac{1000 \text{ mg}}{15 \text{ gr}} \times \dfrac{1 \text{ Gm}}{1000 \text{ mg}} = $ _____ Gm

b. Equivalents: 1 gr = 60 mg, 1000 mg = 1 Gm

Conversion Equation: $5 \text{ gr} \times \dfrac{60 \text{ mg}}{1 \text{ gr}} \times \dfrac{1 \text{ Gm}}{1000 \text{ mg}} = $ _____ Gm

Thus, there may be several routes leading from one starting factor to an equivalent end value. Insofar as possible, it is best to choose the most direct route (i.e., that which requires the fewest conversion factors). Because many of the equivalent relationships, as pointed out before, are *approximations,* the use of additional conversion factors may result in small differences in the end result values. **Therefore, in some instances, the learner may obtain a slightly different answer from the answer key in Appendix C.** Some multiple answers have been included in the key but, obviously, others are possible. When a discrepancy is found, the learner should re-check for accuracy of arithmetic and equivalents. If these are correct, the alternative answer is acceptable. When there is a question as to a safe margin for accuracy, a pharmacist or a drug reference manual should be consulted. In any case, no more than a ten percent difference should occur between the ordered dose of a medication and the amount administered.

Examples: Setting up Conversion Equations

a. How many milligrams are there in 3 grains?
Equivalents: 60 mg = gr 1

Conversion Equation: $\cancel{gr}\,3 \times \dfrac{60\ mg}{\cancel{gr}\,1} =$ _____ mg

b. How many pounds are there in 5 kilograms?
Equivalents: 1 kg = 2.2 lb

Conversion Equation: $5\ \cancel{kg} \times \dfrac{2.2\ lb}{1\ \cancel{kg}} =$ _____ lb

c. How many tablets should the patient receive if the physician ordered 250 mg and each tablet contains 100 mg?
Equivalents: 1 tab = 100 mg

Conversion Equation: $250\ \cancel{mg} \times \dfrac{1\ tab}{100\ \cancel{mg}} =$ _____ tab

d. How many capsules should be administered if the order states gr 2 and the medication label states 60 mg/capsule?
Equivalents: gr 1 = 60 mg, 60 mg = 1 cap

Conversion Equation: $\cancel{gr}\,2 \times \dfrac{60\ \cancel{mg}}{\cancel{gr}\,1} \times \dfrac{1\ cap}{60\ \cancel{mg}} =$ _____ cap

Practice: Setting up Conversion Equations

1. How many ml should be administered if the dose is 250 mg and the label states 500 mg/tsp?
Equivalents:

Conversion Equation:

2. How many minims should the patient receive if the order states 125 mg and the medication strength is 250 mg/5 ml?
Equivalents:

Conversion Equation:

3. How many millimeters are necessary to follow the order of 0.75 Gm if the medication label states 0.5 Gm/ʒi?
Equivalents:

Conversion Equation:

4. How many tablets (scored) will be administered if the ordered dose is gr ⅛ and the tablet strength is 15 mg/tab?
Equivalents:

Conversion Equation:

5. How many milligrams would the patient receive if the order is for 15 ml and the medication strength is 300 mg/tsp?
Equivalents:

Conversion Equation:

(*Note:* See Appendix C for answer key.)

Step III—Solving the Conversion Equation

The third step in the label factor method involves the use of cancellation and simple arithmetic to solve the equation formulated in Step II. If the series of conversion factors has been set up so that corresponding labels are in sequential numerator/denominator positions, the cancellation process will be simplified. Once the labels have been cancelled, the numerical values can likewise be cancelled or reduced to lowest terms, and appropriately multiplied to solve the equation. The resulting answer should be reduced to lowest terms, converted to a decimal, and/or rounded off, as appropriate.

Examples: Solving the Label Factor Equation

a. How many tablets should be administered?
Order: Codeine 60 mg
Label: Codeine gr ½ per tab
Equivalents: 60 mg = gr 1, gr ½ = 1 tab

Conversion Equation: $60 \text{ mg} \times \dfrac{\text{gr } 1}{60 \text{ mg}} \times \dfrac{1 \text{ tab}}{\text{gr } 1/2} = 2 \text{ tab}$

b. How many minims should be administered?
Order: Vistaril 25 mg
Label: Vistaril (hydroxyzine HCl) 100 mg/2 ml
Equivalents: 100 mg = 2 ml, 1 ml = 15 m

Conversion Equation: $25 \text{ mg} \times \dfrac{2 \text{ ml}}{100 \text{ mg}} \times \dfrac{15 \text{ m}}{1 \text{ ml}} = 7.5 \text{ m} = 8 \text{ m}$

(*Note:* Refer to Appendix A for basic arithmetic review.)

Practice: Solving Conversion Equations

1. **Order:** Lanoxin 0.250 mg
   Label: Lanoxin (digoxin) 0.125 mg/tab
   Question: How many tablets should the patient receive? _____
   Equivalents:

   Conversion Equation:

2. **Order:** Nembutal gr ½
   Label: Nembutal (pentobarbital) 30 mg/cap
   Question: How many capsules should the nurse give? _____
   Equivalents:

   Conversion Equation:

3. **Order:** Tolinase 250 mg
   Label: Tolinase (tolazamide) 0.5 Gm/tab (scored)
   Question: How many tablets should be administered? _____
   Equivalents:

   Conversion Equation:

4. **Order:** Morphine Sulphate gr ⅙
   Label: Morphine Sulphate gr ¼ per 20 m
   Question: How many ml should be administered? (*Note:* Carry
   answer to three places and round to two.) _____
   Equivalents:

   Conversion Equation:

5. **Order:** Atropine gr ¹⁄₁₀₀
   Label: Atropine gr ¹⁄₁₅₀ per ml
   Question: How many minims should be administered? _____
   Equivalents:

   Conversion Equation:

6. **Order:** Chloral hydrate elixir 1 Gm
   Label: Chloral hydrate elixir gr 7 ½ per 5 ml
   Question: How many ml will equal this dose? _____
   Equivalents:

   Conversion Equation:

7. **Order:** Riopan 10 ml
   Label: Riopan (magaldrate) 400 mg/tsp
   Question: How many mg will be contained in this dose? _____
   Equivalents:

   Conversion Equation:

8. **Order:** Ceclor 200 mg
   Label: Ceclor (cefaclor) 125 mg/5 ml
   Question: How many ml must be administered? _____
   Equivalents:

   Conversion Equation:

9. **Order:** Dilantin 30 Pediatric Suspension 75 mg
   Label: Dilantin 30 (phenytoin sodium) Pediatric Suspension 30 mg/
      5 ml
   Question: How many ml should be administered? _____
   Equivalents:

   Conversion Equation:

10. **Order:** Phenobarbital 90 mg
    Label: Phenobarbital gr 1 ½ per tab
    Question: How many tablets should be given? _____
    Equivalents:

    Conversion Equation:

(*Note:* See Appendix C for answer key)

The learner who is having difficulty solving equations should seek remedial assistance before proceeding further.

Important Points to Remember

1. Be sure the starting factor is the first item and the answer label is the last item in the conversion equation.
2. Use only conversion factors that have a 1 : 1 relationship.
3. Set up the conversion equation so that cancellable labels appear in consecutive numerator/denominator.
4. When solving the conversion equation:

   ■ cancel labels first.
   ■ reduce numbers to lowest terms.
   ■ multiply/divide to solve the equation.
   ■ reduce answer to lowest terms, convert to decimal, and/or round off.

Accuracy and Accountability

The learner is cautioned against blind reliance on any formula, particularly when its use has become familiar and automatic. The application of common sense and reasonable prudence will help prevent medication errors due to either carelessness or inaccuracy in determining equivalents and solving conversion equations.

Although the level of arithmetic required to solve nearly all label factor problems is almost elementary, math errors do occur. This means that it is essential to double-check the computation, even if a calculator is used.

To this end, the learner should develop the habit of carefully inspecting the information given in every problem and seeking simple benchmarks relative to the anticipated answer. For example, should it be less than or more than one tablet, grain, or milliliter? What is a typical and reasonable amount of solution for an intravenous, an intramuscular, or an oral medication? Extremely large numbers should be suspect: answers such as 12 tablets po, 850 gtt/min IV, 16 ml IM should be questioned as *illogical* and *unreasonable*. When there is any doubt as to the accuracy of a computation, a drug reference should be consulted to be sure the answer is consistent with the recommended range of dosage for that particular drug. An additional resource for verification is the registered pharmacist.

Medication errors constitute one of the greatest areas of risk for which health-care providers can be vulnerable to negligence or malpractice litigation. Although it is hoped that the use of a single and consistent approach to calculating medication dosages will help prevent medication errors, it must be emphasized that any method or formula is only as safe as the individual using it.

Remember: The final step in solving any problem, of course, is to ask whether the answer is reasonable. Common sense and common caution are prerequisites to use of the label factor method in clinical calculations.

The Metric System of Measurement

•••

Objectives
Upon completion of this unit of study you should be able to:
- *Identify the three basic units of measurement in the metric system: gram, liter, and meter.*
- *List metric abbreviations and prefixes commonly used in drug computations.*
- *Compare various metric units in relation to length, weight, and volume.*
- *Apply the label factor method to conversion of equal values within the metric system.*

Basic Units
The basic units of measurement in the metric system are the gram as the unit of weight, the liter as the unit of volume, and the meter as the unit of length, Table 2-1. The main feature of the metric system is that each of the basic units may be divided into decimal values or expanded into multiples of ten by the use of standard prefixes, Table 2-2.

Metric Abbreviations
The basic units gram, liter, and meter are most commonly divided into certain units for clinical calculations, as seen in Table 2-3.

Metric Notation
In the metric system, quantities are written with the number preceding the unit. Arabic whole numbers and decimals are used rather than Roman numerals or fractions, Table 2-4.

Comparing Metric Units
When converting metric values, make use of the obvious principle: "It takes many small units to equal a large unit." For example, in Table 2-5, it can be seen that a milligram is 0.001 gram and is a small unit. It would take 1,000 milligrams to equal one gram, Figure 2-1. However, a kilogram is a large unit. It takes 1,000 grams to equal one kilogram. Similarly, a milliliter is 0.001 L and is a small unit, Table 2-6. It takes 1,000 ml to equal one liter, Figure 2-2. Finally, the small unit, millimeter, equals one

Table 2-1. METRIC UNITS

TYPE	UNIT
weight (mass)	gram
volume (liquid)	liter
length	meter

Table 2-2. METRIC PREFIXES

SMALL UNITS	LARGE UNITS
deci = 0.1	deka = 10
centi = 0.01	hecto = 100
milli = 0.001	kilo = 1,000
micro = 0.000001	mega = 1,000,000

Table 2-3. METRIC ABBREVIATIONS

TYPE	UNIT	ABBREVIATIONS USED IN THIS TEXT	ALTERNATIVE ACCEPTABLE ABBREVIATIONS
weight	gram	Gm	gm, g
	milligram	mg	mgm
	microgram	mcg	μg
	kilogram	kg	Kg
volume	liter	L	l
	milliliter*	ml	cc
	minim	m	ℳ
length	meter	M	m
	centimeter	cm	
	millimeter	mm	

* A milliliter is a small unit of volume frequently used in dispensing medication. It has the same volume as a cubic centimeter (cc). The abbreviations cc and ml may be used interchangeably.

Table 2-4. METRIC NOTATION

QUANTITY	NOTATION
1 gram	1 Gm
60 milligrams	60 mg
3 liters	3 L
500 milliliters	500 ml
10 meters	10 M
150 centimeters	150 cm

Table 2-5.   METRIC UNITS OF WEIGHT

MANY SMALL UNITS EQUAL ONE LARGE UNIT

1mg = 0.001 Gm; 1,000 mg = 1 Gm
1 mcg (μg) = 0.000001 Gm; 1,000,000 mcg (μg) = 1 Gm
1 mcg (μg) = 0.000001 Gm; 1,000 mcg (μg) = 1 mg
1 Gm = 0.001 kg; 1,000 Gm = 1 kg

Table 2-6.   METRIC UNITS OF VOLUME

MANY SMALL UNITS EQUAL ONE LARGE UNIT

1 ml = 0.001 L; 1,000 ml = 1 L

Table 2-7.   METRIC UNITS OF LENGTH

MANY SMALL UNITS EQUAL ONE LARGE UNIT

1 mm = 0.001 M; 1,000 mm = 1 M
1 cm = 0.01 M; 100 cm = 1 M

---

one thousandth of a meter, Table 2-7. It takes 10 millimeters to equal 1 centimeter and 100 centimeters to equal 1 meter, Figure 2-3.

Obviously, there are many more divisions and multiples of the basic metric units possible. Tables 2-1 to 2-7 contain the quantities most frequently used in clinical calculations of dosages and measurements; these relationships should be memorized.

Converting Units Within the Metric System

Using the previously memorized prefixes and relationships as equivalent values, complete the Practice following the steps used in the examples.

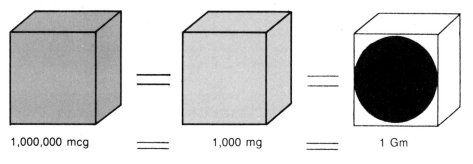

1,000,000 mcg —— 1,000 mg —— 1 Gm

Figure 2-1

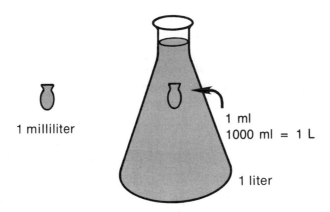

Figure 2-2

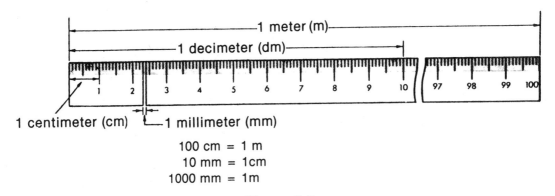

100 cm = 1 m
10 mm = 1cm
1000 mm = 1m

Figure 2-3

(*Note:* Carry each answer to two decimal places and round to nearest tenth.)

Examples:

   a. Convert 0.16 centimeters to millimeters.
     Starting Factor   Answer Label
        0.16 cm   mm
     Equivalents: 1 cm = 0.01 M; 1 mm = 0.001 M

   Conversion Equation: $0.16 \ \cancel{cm} \times \dfrac{0.01 \ \cancel{M}}{1 \ \cancel{cm}} \times \dfrac{1 \ mm}{0.001 \ \cancel{M}} = 1.6 \ mm$

b. Convert 240 micrograms to milligrams.

   Starting Factor   Answer Label

      240 mcg   mg

   Equivalents: 1 mg = 1,000 mcg

$$\text{Conversion Equation: } 240 \text{ mcg} \times \frac{1 \text{ mg}}{1,000 \text{ mcg}} = 0.2 \text{ mg}$$

c. Convert 375 milligrams to grams.

   Equivalents: 1,000 mg = 1 Gm; 1 mg = 0.001 Gm

$$\text{Conversion Equation: } 375 \text{ mg} \times \frac{1 \text{ Gm}}{1,000 \text{ mg}} = 0.4 \text{ Gm}$$

OR

$$375 \text{ mg} \times \frac{0.001 \text{ Gm}}{1 \text{ mg}} = 0.4 \text{ Gm}$$

d. Convert 75 grams to kilograms.

   Equivalents: 1,000 Gm = 1 kg; 1 Gm = 0.001 kg

$$\text{Conversion Equation: } 75 \text{ Gm} \times \frac{1 \text{ kg}}{1,000 \text{ Gm}} = 0.1 \text{ kg}$$

OR

$$75 \text{ Gm} \times \frac{0.001 \text{ kg}}{1 \text{ Gm}} = 0.1 \text{ kg}$$

Practice: Convert Within the Metric System

1. 3225 ml to L

2. 375 mg to Gm

3. 2000 Gm to kg

4. 5000 mcg to mg

5. 29 cm to M

6. 0.75 L to ml

7. 0.22 Gm to mg

8. 2.5 kg to Gm

9. 25 mm to cm

10. 12 mg to mcg

(*Note:* See Appendix C for answer key.)

The Apothecaries System of Measurement

●●

Objectives

Upon completion of this unit of study you should be able to:
- *Identify the four basic units of measurement in the apothecaries system: grain, minim, fluid dram, fluid ounce.*
- *List apothecaries abbreviations and symbols commonly used in drug computations.*
- *Compare various apothecaries units in relation to weight and volume.*
- *Apply the label factor method to conversion of equal values within the apothecaries system.*

Although the apothecaries system of measurement is being replaced by the metric, the former system is still commonly enough used in writing prescriptions and medication orders that the nurse should be familiar with it, particularly its symbols and abbreviations, Table 3-1.

Basic Units and Abbreviations

In the apothecaries system, the grain is the basic unit of weight and the minim, fluid dram, and fluid ounce are the basic units of volume. The latter two usually are shortened to dram and ounce. Although dry weights can be measured in drams and ounces, they are rarely so measured for medication computations. Therefore, when these terms are used in medication orders or calculations in this text, they refer to fluid volume. An exception to this rule is in the preparation of percentage solutions, which will be illustrated in Appendix B. Additionally, the pint and quart are units of volume that are rarely used in the administration of medications.

When body weight is required for calculation of dosage, the pound unit is used. In the traditional apothecaries system, the pound consists of 12 (dry weight) ounces; however, it is common practice in this country to employ the 16 ounce avoirdupois pound for dry weights. Therefore, any

Table 3-1. BASIC APOTHECARIES UNITS

TYPE	UNIT	ABBREVIATION
weight	grain	gr
	pound (16 oz)	lb
volume	minim	m
	dram	dr or ȝ
	ounce	oz or ℥
	pint	pt or 0
	quart	qt

computation involving conversions of pound units in this text "implies" use of the 16 ounce pound.

It is important to note the difference between the dram and ounce symbols, as seen in Table 3-1. The dram, which is a smaller amount, has one less loop than the ounce symbol, which represents the larger amount. **Confusion of these two symbols can result in a serious medication error.**

Apothecaries Notation

When writing quantities in the apothecaries system, the number *follows* the unit, in contrast to the metric system. For small numbers up to 40, lower-case Roman numerals are used; for large or complex numbers above 40, Arabic numbers may be substituted.

Table 3-2 shows examples of traditional apothecaries notations. However, in the clinical setting, the practitioner frequently will encounter apothecaries notations written in the metric form, that is, Arabic numbers preceding the unit. The learner should become familiar with both methods of apothecaries notations; they will be used interchangeably in this text.

Table 3-2. APOTHECARIES NOTATION

QUANTITY	NOTATION
$1/10$ grain	gr $1/10$
1 grain	gr i
1 $1/2$ grains	gr iss
10 grains	gr x
15 minims	m xv
150 minims	m 150
2 $1/2$ ounces	iss

Note, in particular, the use of the abbreviation s̄s̄. Used alone, this symbol means ½; when larger quantities are denoted: 1 ½, 2 ½, the appropriate numeral is placed to the left of the symbol.

Practice: Write the Abbreviation for Each of the Following:

1. dram (symbol)   = _____
2. grain   = _____
3. minim   = _____
4. one half   = _____
5. ounce (symbol)   = _____

(*Note:* See Appendix C for answer key.)

Comparing Apothecaries Units

In comparing apothecaries values, the learner should keep in mind, as with metric units, that many small units equal one large unit. For example, a minim is a small amount; it takes 60 minims to equal one dram, Figure 3-1. However, a quart is a large unit; it would take 256 drams to equal one quart, Table 3-3.

Converting Units Within the Apothecaries System

Using the apothecaries equivalents, complete the Practice following the steps used in the examples.

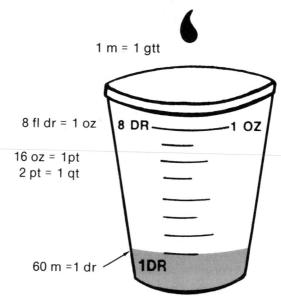

1 m = 1 gtt

8 fl dr = 1 oz   8 DR ——————— 1 OZ

16 oz = 1pt
2 pt = 1 qt

60 m =1 dr   1DR

Figure 3-1

Table 3-3. APOTHECARIES FLUID UNITS

60 m = 1 dr (ℨ)
8 dr = 1 oz (℥)
16 oz = 1 pt (O)
2 pt = 1 qt

Examples:

a. Convert 30 minims to drams.
   Starting Factor   Answer Label
       30 m   dr
   Equivalents: 60 m = 1 dr

   Conversion Equation: $30 \text{ m} \times \dfrac{1 \text{ dr}}{60 \text{ m}} = \frac{1}{2} \text{ dr}$

b. Convert 64 drams to pints.
   Starting Factor   Answer Label
       64 dr   pt
   Equivalents: 8 dr = 1 oz, 16 oz = 1 pt

   Conversion Equation: $64 \text{ dr} \times \dfrac{1 \text{ oz}}{8 \text{ dr}} \times \dfrac{1 \text{ pt}}{16 \text{ oz}} = \frac{1}{2} \text{ pt}$

c. Convert 55 ounces to quarts.
   Starting Factor   Answer Label
       55 oz   qt
   Equivalents: 32 oz = 1 qt

   Conversion Equation: $55 \text{ oz} \times \dfrac{1 \text{ qt}}{32 \text{ oz}} = 1 \, ^7/_{10} \text{ qt}$

d. Convert 4 drams to ounces.
   Starting Factor   Answer Label
       4 dr   oz
   Equivalents: 8 dr = 1 oz

   Conversion Equation: $4 \text{ dr} \times \dfrac{1 \text{ oz}}{8 \text{ dr}} = \frac{1}{2} \text{ oz}$

e. Convert pints iss to ℨ.
   Starting Factor   Answer Label
       1 ½ pt   oz
   Equivalents: 1 pt = 16 oz, 1 oz = 8 dr

   Conversion Equation: $1 \frac{1}{2} \text{ pt} \times \dfrac{16 \text{ oz}}{1 \text{ pt}} \times \dfrac{8 \text{ dr}}{1 \text{ oz}} = 192 \text{ dr}$

Practice: Convert Within the Apothecaries System

1. 55 oz to qt

2. 4 dr to oz

3. pt i̅s̅s̅ to ℥

4. 30 m to ℨ

5. 2 ml to ℨ

6. 1 ¼ oz to ℨ

7. 120 m to ℥

8. 2 pts to dr

9. 3 ½ lb to oz

10. 62.4 oz to lb

(*Note:* See Appendix C for answer key.)

The Household System of Measurement

••

Objectives

Upon completion of this unit of study you should be able to:

- *Identify the units of measurement in the household system: drops, teaspoons, tablespoons, cups, and glasses.*
- *List household abbreviations commonly used in drug computations.*
- *Compare various household units in relation to volume.*
- *Apply the label factor method to conversion of equal values within the household system.*

Household Units

The household system of measurement involves the use of drops, spoons, cups, and glasses, Table 4-1. These units, which are derived from household measuring utensils, are not very precise. For example, the size of a drop of fluid will vary depending on the temperature, the composition of the fluid, and the size of the opening from which the drop emerges. The use of cups and spoons as measuring apparatus cannot compare to the accuracy of graduates and syringes as used with the metric system.

Household units are used primarily in the administration of external preparations such as baths, soaks, gargles, enemas, compresses, and disinfectants. They also are used in measuring oral fluid intake where a high degree of accuracy is not necessary. These units and their approximate equivalents are listed in Table 4-2.

> **Remember: A rule of thumb for making an 0.85 percent or 0.9 percent normal saline solution for gargles, enemas, etc., is to use one teaspoon of salt to one pint of water.**

Table 4-1.   HOUSEHOLD UNITS

TYPE	UNIT	ABBREVIATION
weight	ounce	oz
	pound (16 oz)	lb
volume	drop	gtt
	teaspoon	tsp or t
	tablespoon	tbsp or T
	ounce	oz
	cup/glass	c/gl
	pint	pt
	quart	qt
length	inch	in
	foot	ft

Table 4-2.   HOUSEHOLD EQUIVALENTS

$$60 \text{ gtt} = 1 \text{ tsp}$$
$$3 \text{ tsp} = 1 \text{ tbsp} = \frac{1}{2} \text{ oz}$$
$$2 \text{ tbsp} = 1 \text{ oz}$$
$$6 \text{ oz} = 1 \text{ teacup}$$
$$8 \text{ oz} = 1 \text{ glass or measuring cup}$$
$$16 \text{ oz} = 1 \text{ pt}$$

The more commonly used units should be memorized, because of their frequency of use in the situations mentioned previously.

Household Notation

In the household system, quantities are written in the same manner as in the metric system; the number (quantity) precedes the unit and Arabic whole numbers are used. Fractions or decimals may be used for quantities which are portions of whole numbers, Table 4-3.

Practice: Write the Abbreviations for Each of the Following:

1. drop   = _____
2. gallon   = _____
3. pint   = _____
4. tablespoon = _____
5. teaspoon   = _____

(*Note:* See Appendix C for answer key.)

Comparing Household Units

Figure 4-1 illustrates the progression of the various units of volume in the household system of measurement.

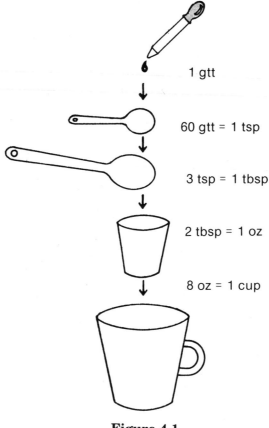

1 gtt

60 gtt = 1 tsp

3 tsp = 1 tbsp

2 tbsp = 1 oz

8 oz = 1 cup

Figure 4-1

Table 4-3.   HOUSEHOLD NOTATION

QUANTITY	NOTATION
1 drop	1 gtt
3 teaspoons	3 tsp
8 ounces	8 oz
2 pints	2 pt

Converting Units Within the Household System

Using the relationships given as equivalent values, complete the Practice following the steps used in the examples. (*Note:* Carry each answer to two decimal places and round to nearest tenth.)

Examples:

a. Convert 16 tablespoons to cups.

Starting Factor   Answer Label
    16 tbsp   cup

Equivalents: 2 tbsp = 1 oz; 8 oz = 1 cup

Conversion Equation: $16 \text{ tbsp} \times \dfrac{1 \text{ oz}}{2 \text{ tbsp}} \times \dfrac{1 \text{ cup}}{8 \text{ oz}} = 1 \text{ cup}$

b. Convert 5 ounces to teaspoons.

Starting Factor   Answer Label
    5 oz   tsp

Equivalents: 1 oz = 6 tsp

Conversion Equation: $5 \text{ oz} \times \dfrac{6 \text{ tsp}}{1 \text{ oz}} = 30 \text{ tsp}$

Practice: Convert Within the Household System

1. 1 glass to tsp

2. 2 gal to oz

3. 4 qt to cups

4. 68 in to ft

5. 4 tbsp to oz

6. 6 tbsp to tsp

7. 22 pts to gal

8. 2.6 lb to oz

9. 50 tsp to oz

10. 1 teacup to tbsp

(*Note:* See Appendix C for answer key.)

Conversion of Metric, Apothecaries, and Household Units

••

Objectives

Upon completion of this unit of study you should be able to:
- *List approximate equivalent values among the three systems of measurement: metric, apothecaries, and household.*
- *Apply the label factor method to conversions of equivalent values among these systems of measurement.*

It is essential that nurses be able to convert accurately among the various systems of measurement, because medication orders often are written in one system and dispensed in another.

Having memorized the basic units and relationships within the metric, apothecaries, and household systems, the learner is now ready to apply the label factor method to conversions among these systems. Table 5-1 illustrates the equivalent relationships among the metric, apothecaries, and household systems. Also study Figures 5-1, 5-2, and 5-3 to visualize these relationships.

Self-Quiz—Equivalents

A. Fill in the blanks
   1. 60 mg = _____ gr
   2. 15 gr = _____ Gm
   3. 1 Gm = _____ mg
   4. 1 kg   = _____ Gm
   5. 1 kg   = _____ lb
   6. 1 m   = _____ gtt
   7. 1 L   = _____ ml
   8. 1 in   = _____ cm

9. 1 M   = _____ in
10. 1 tbsp = _____ oz

B. Match equivalent amounts

_____1. 1 ml   a. 1 oz
_____2. 1 tsp   b. 4 dr
_____3. 1 cup   c. 5 ml
_____4. 15 ml   d. 15 m
_____5. 30 ml   e. 250 ml
                              f. 500 ml

(*Note:* See Appendix C for answer key.)

Table 5-1. APPROXIMATE EQUIVALENTS AMONG METRIC, APOTHECARIES, AND HOUSEHOLD SYSTEMS

METRIC		APOTHECARIES		HOUSEHOLD
Dry				
60 mg	=	1 gr		
1 Gm	=	15 gr		
15 Gm	=	4 dr	=	1 tbsp (3 tsp)
30 Gm	=	1 oz (8 dr)	=	1 oz (2 tbsp)
		16 oz	=	1 lb (avoirdupois)
1 kg			=	2.2 lb
Liquid				
		1 m	=	1 gtt
1 ml	=	15 m	=	15 gtt
4 ml	=	1 dr		
5 ml	=	75 m	=	1 tsp
15 ml	=	4 dr	=	1 tbsp (3 tsp)
30 ml	=	1 oz (8 dr)	=	1 fl oz (2 tbsp)
500 ml	=	16 oz (1 pt)	=	16 oz (1 pt or 2 cups)
1000 ml	=	32 oz (1 qt)	=	32 oz (1 qt)
Length				
2.5 cm			=	1 in
1 M			=	39.4 in

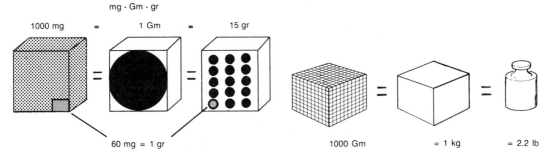

Figure 5-1

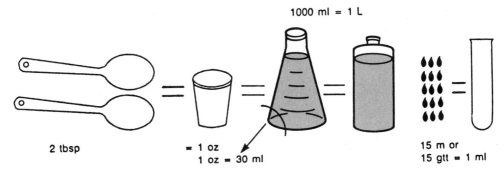

Figure 5-2

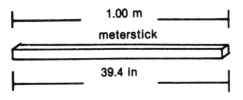

1 m = 39.4 in

Figure 5-3

Conversion From One System to Another
Examples:

a. Convert 5 Gm to gr

   Starting Factor   Answer Label
       5 Gm   gr

   Equivalents: 1 Gm = 15 gr

   Conversion Equation: $5 \text{ Gm} \times \dfrac{15 \text{ gr}}{1 \text{ Gm}} = 75 \text{ gr}$

b. Convert 5.4 lb to kg

   Starting Factor   Answer Label
       5.4 lb   kg

   Equivalents: 1 kg = 2.2 lb

   Conversion Equation: $5.4 \text{ lb} \times \dfrac{1 \text{ kg}}{2.2 \text{ lb}} = 2.5 \text{ kg}$

c. Convert gr 45 to Gm

   Starting Factor   Answer Label
       gr 45   _____ Gm

   Equivalents: gr 15 = 1 Gm

   Conversion Equation: $\text{gr } 45 \times \dfrac{1 \text{ Gm}}{\text{gr } 15} = 3 \text{ Gm}$

d. Convert 54 kg to lb

   Starting Factor   Answer Label
       54 kg   _____ lb

   Equivalents: 2.2 lb = 1 kg

   Conversion Equation: $54 \text{ kg} \times \dfrac{2.2 \text{ lb}}{1 \text{ kg}} = 118.8 \text{ lb}$

e. Convert 16 ml to dr

   Starting Factor   Answer Label
       16 ml   _____ dr

   Equivalents: 4 ml = 1 dr

   Conversion Equation: $16 \text{ ml} \times \dfrac{1 \text{ dr}}{4 \text{ ml}} = 4 \text{ dr}$

f. Convert 8 oz to ml

   Starting Factor   Answer Label
       8 oz   _____ ml

   Equivalents: 1 oz = 30 ml

Conversion Equation: $8 \text{ o̶z̶} \times \dfrac{30 \text{ ml}}{1 \text{ o̶z̶}} = 240 \text{ ml}$

g. Convert 480 ml to oz
   Starting Factor   Answer Label
       480 ml   _____ oz
   Equivalents: 30 ml = 1 oz

   Conversion Equation: $480 \text{ m̶l̶} \times \dfrac{1 \text{ oz}}{30 \text{ m̶l̶}} = 16 \text{ oz}$

h. Convert gr 2 ½ to mg
   Starting Factor   Answer Label
       gr 2 ½   _____ mg
   Equivalents: gr 1 = 60 mg

   Conversion Equation: $\text{g̶r̶ } 2 \text{ ½} \times \dfrac{60 \text{ mg}}{\text{g̶r̶}1} = 150 \text{ mg}$

i. Convert 300 mg to gr
   Starting Factor   Answer Label
       300 mg   gr _____
   Equivalents: 60 mg = gr 1

   Conversion Equation: $300 \text{ m̶g̶} \times \dfrac{\text{gr } 1}{60 \text{ m̶g̶}} = \text{gr } 5$

j. Convert 10 ml to tsp
   Starting Factor   Answer Label
       10 ml   _____ tsp
   Equivalents: 5 ml = 1 tsp

   Conversion Equation: $10 \text{ m̶l̶} \times \dfrac{1 \text{ tsp}}{5 \text{ m̶l̶}} = 2 \text{ tsp}$

Practice: (Carry each answer to two decimal places and round to the nearest tenth.)
   1. 2.5 pts to ml

   2. 40 kg to lb

3. 600 ml to cups

4. 2 tsp to ml

5. gr $\overline{ss}$ to mg

6. ℥ 50 to kg

7. m xx to ml

8. ℥ iv to tbsp

9. 0.6 L to ℥

10. 2 Gm to gr

11. ℈ iss̄ to gtt

12. 5 ml to m

13. 120 mg to gr

14. 10 gtt to ml

15. 12.5 ml to tsp

16. 1 ½ tbsp to ml

17. 2 cups to ml

18. 6 tsp to ʒ

19. 120 gr to Gm

20. 157 lb to kg

21. gr 3 to mg

22. 3 ml to m

23. 5.2 kg to lb

24. 120 mm to cm

25. 60 cm to in

26. 0.5 pt to 3

27. 90 mg to gr

28. 5.5 Gm to gr

29. 60 ml to tbsp

30. 5 gr to mg

(*Note:* See Appendix C for answer key.)

Calculation of Oral Medications

••

Objectives

Upon completion of this unit of study you should be able to:
- *Identify various forms of oral medications.*
- *Read dosage calibrations on a medicine cup, dropper, and syringe.*
- *Read drug labels to obtain information about specific drugs administered orally.*
- *Demonstrate knowledge of the appropriate method of rounding off doses when administering oral medications.*
- *Apply the label factor method to clinical calculations involving oral medications.*

Oral Medications

Medications that are administered by mouth and absorbed via the gastrointestinal tract are known as po (per os, by mouth) drugs. It is necessary to become familiar with this abbreviation to administer these drugs by the correct route, which should be designated as po (or o) in the medication order.

A variation of the oral route is called the *sublingual route,* whereby medication is placed under the tongue for absorption via the mucous membrane into the circulatory system. This route is designated by the abbreviation sl in the medication order. When medication is ordered to be administered via the buccal route, it is placed between the cheek and gum for similar absorption. Neither sublingual nor buccal medications should be chewed or swallowed whole and, as a rule, are not followed by water.

It is necessary to recognize the various forms in which oral medications are dispensed and to understand how to read labels of medication containers, as well as calibrations on equipment used to dispense liquid medications.

Figure 6-1 illustrates a variety of oral medication forms:

■ Tablets—contain a powdered drug compressed into a tablet. Tablets come in various shapes and may be half-scored or quarter-scored. They

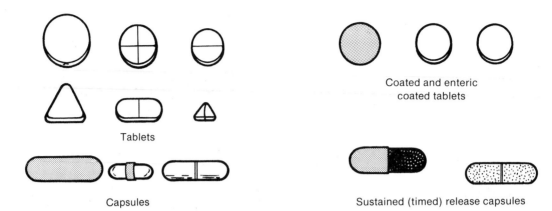

Figure 6-1   Oral medication forms

may be broken or crushed and placed in food for patients who have difficulty swallowing.

■ Coated tablets—covered with a flavored coating to facilitate swallowing and disguise taste. They cannot be divided and should not be crushed.

■ Enteric coated—covered with a coating that delays dissolution and absorption until tablet reaches the small intestine. They cannot be divided and should not be crushed.

■ Capsules—contain a drug enclosed in a gelatin container to conceal taste. May be opened and contents placed in food, unless this is contra-indicated by desired action of the drug.

■ Sustained-release capsules or tablets—drug granules coated to dissolve at different times to provide for continuous release of drug over an extended time period. (Also called timed-release capsules, spansules, tempules, or capulets.) Must never be opened or broken apart before administering.

■ Liquids—dispensed as elixirs, syrups, suspensions, or solutions.

The Medicine Cup

The most common type of container used for dispensing fluid drugs is the medicine cup, made of glass or plastic, Figure 6-2. It usually is calibrated in one or more of the three measuring systems: metric, apothecaries, and household.

When a solution is poured into a medicine cup, capillary attraction causes the fluid in contact with the cup to be drawn upward and the surface of the solution becomes concave. The curved surface is called the

Medicine Cup

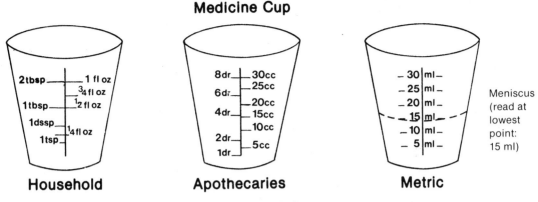

Figure 6-2 Medicine cup

meniscus and the reading of the dose must be made at the lowest point of the meniscus when the cup is held at eye level.

Note that the smallest amounts for which most medicine cups are calibrated are 1 dram, 1 teaspoon, or 5 milliliters. When measuring smaller amounts, it is recommended that the medication be drawn up into a syringe, which facilitates a more accurate measurement. Some liquid medications are premeasured for oral administration in a single-dose syringe.

When pills, tablets, or capsules are being dispensed, they may be placed in a plastic medicine cup or in a small paper (souffle) cup, depending on hospital policy. Many such medications are wrapped individually and should be opened at the bedside just prior to administration.

Rounding Off

When Administering Tablets

■ Scored tablets may be broken in half or quarters in order to obtain as exact a dose as possible, Figure 6-1.

Example: If calculated dose is: 1.5 tablets, give 1 ½ tablets

1.25 tablets, give 1 ¼ tablets

1.75 tablets, give 1 ¾ tablets

■ If tablets are not scored, round up or down to the nearest tablet.

Example: If calculated dose is: 1.1–1.4 tablets, give 1 tablet

1.5–1.9 tablets, give 2 tablets

(*Note:* This is a very inaccurate method and should be used only when an alternative form (e.g., liquid) of the medication is not available. Check with the pharmacist regarding alternate dosage forms.)

■ Capsules, spansules, and enteric coated tablets cannot be divided. These dosages should also be rounded to the nearest whole number.

When Administering Liquids

■ If measuring in milliliters, carry the calculation to two decimal places and round to the nearest tenth. If the calculated dose is an even multiple of 5, it may be measured in the medicine cup. Any dosage that is not an even multiple of 5 should be measured using a syringe as this permits accurate measurement of small amounts, including tenths of milliliters, Figure 6-3.

Example: If calculated dose is: 2.3 ml, draw up entire amount in syringe

5 ml, measure in medicine cup

12.7 ml, pour 10 ml into medicine cup, draw up 2.7 ml into syringe, and add to medication in cup

■ If measuring in teaspoons or tablespoons, carry the calculation to two decimal places and round to the nearest tenth. If the calculated dose is an exact teaspoon or tablespoon, it may be measured in the medicine cup. Any dosage that is not an exact teaspoon or tablespoon should be converted to milliliters and measured as above, using a syringe. This is a more accurate method than converting milliliters to drops.

■ Liquid medications often are dispensed with a dropper attached to the bottle cap. This dropper usually is calibrated in milliliters (e.g., 0.1

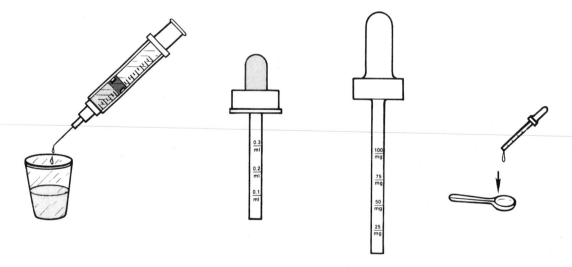

Figure 6-3

ml, 0.2 ml) or by actual dosage (e.g., 75 mg, 100 mg), thus facilitating accurate measurement of the medication, Figure 6-3.

■ Medications that are ordered in drops (household system) can be drawn up into a dropper and the required number of drops placed in a spoon or medicine cup for administration, Figure 6-3.

Reading Labels and Calculating Dosage

All medication containers are labeled as to their contents and directions for use. Individuals administering medications must be able to read and understand the information given on the label. This information includes:

■ Name of drug: Trade name—the brand name; the registered trademark assigned by the manufacturer; usually followed by ®. Generic name (by law this must appear on all drug labels)—the official name assigned to a drug; the name under which it is licensed. Drugs that have been in use for many years may thereafter be manufactured and sold under the generic name, eliminating the need for a brand name. Therefore, if only one name appears on a drug label, it is the generic name.

■ Dosage strength: Amount or concentration of the drug—per vial, ampule, ml, tablet, capsule, etc. This may be written in more than one system of measurement (e.g., metric, apothecaries).

■ Name of manufacturer

Some labels may also indicate:

■ Form: Liquid—ml, oz, etc. Solid-tablet, capsule, powder, etc. (not always indicated on the label).

■ Expiration date: How long the medication (usually liquid) will remain stable or potent.

■ Total amount per container: Total volume, if liquid; total number, if solid. It is important not to confuse this number or quantity with the dosage strength of the drug.

■ Directions for administering (or storing): mixing, reconstituting, shaking, refrigerating, etc.

Examples: Reading Labels

Figure 6-4

1. Trade Name: Lanoxin
2. Generic Name: Digoxin
3. Dosage Strength: 125 mcg (μg), same as 0.125 mg per tablet
4. Form: Tablet
5. Manufacturer's Name: Burroughs Wellcome Co.
6. Expiration Date: 12/89

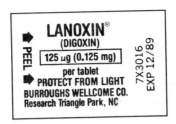

Figure 6-4   *(Courtesy Burroughs Wellcome Co.)*

7. **Order:** Lanoxin 0.250 mg po
   How many tablets should the patient receive?

   Starting Factor   Answer Label
      0.250 mg   tab
   Equivalent: 0.125 mg = 1 tab

   Conversion Equation: $0.250 \text{ mg} \times \dfrac{1 \text{ tab}}{0.125 \text{ mg}} = 2 \text{ tab}$

Figure 6-5

1. Trade Name: None
2. Generic Name: Potassium Chloride
3. Dosage Strength: 300 mg (5 gr)
4. Form: Enteric coated tablets
5. Manufacturer's Name: Lilly

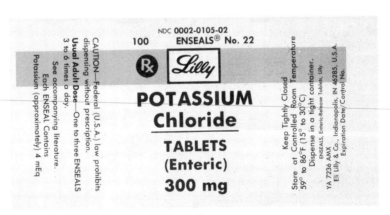

Figure 6-5   *(Courtesy Eli Lilly & Co.)*

6. **Order:** Potassium Chloride gr 10 po
   How many tablets should the patient receive?
   Starting Factor   Answer Label
       gr 10   tab
   Equivalent: gr 5= 1 tab

   Conversion Equation: $\cancel{gr}\,10 \times \dfrac{1\,\text{tab}}{\cancel{gr}\,5} = 2\text{ tab}$

   OR

   Equivalents: gr 1 = 60 mg, 300 mg = 1 tab

   Conversion Equation: $\cancel{gr}\,10 \times \dfrac{60\,\cancel{mg}}{\cancel{gr}\,1} \times \dfrac{1\,\text{tab}}{300\,\cancel{mg}} = 2\text{ tab}$

Practice: Reading Labels

A. Figure 6-6
   1. Trade Name: _____
   2. Generic Name: _____
   3. Dosage Strength: _____
   4. Form: _____
   5. Manufacturer's Name: _____
   6. **Order:** Inderal LA 80 mg po
      How many capsules should be administered? _____
   7. **Order:** Inderal LA 160 mg po
      How many capsules should be administered? _____

B. Figure 6-7
   1. Trade Name: _____
   2. Generic Name: _____
   3. Dosage Strength: _____
   4. Form: _____
   5. Manufacturer's Name: _____
   6. **Order:** KCl 15 mEq po
      How many ml should the patient receive? _____
   7. **Order:** KCl 10 mEq po
      How many ml should the patient receive? _____

C. Figure 6-8
   1. Trade Name: _____
   2. Generic Name: _____
   3. Dosage Strength: _____
   4. Form: _____
   5. Manufacturer's Name: _____

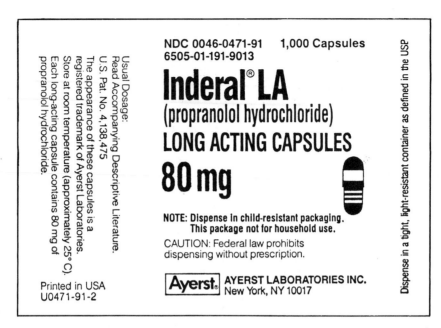

Figure 6-6   *(Courtesy Wyeth-Ayerst Laboratories, Inc.)*

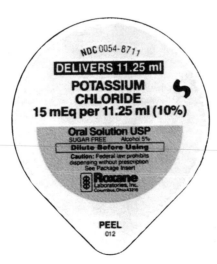

Figure 6-7   *(Courtesy Roxane Laboratories, Inc.)*

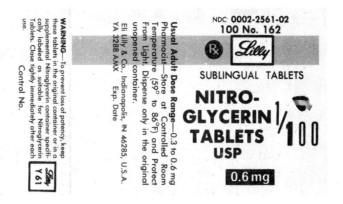

Figure 6-8   *(Courtesy Eli Lilly & Co.)*

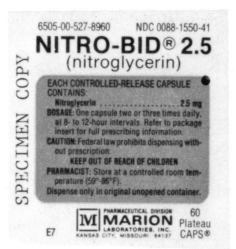

Figure 6-9   *(Courtesy Marion Laboratories, Inc.)*

D. Figure 6-9
    1.   Trade Name: _____
    2.   Generic Name: _____
    3.   Dosage Strength: _____
    4.   Form: _____
    5.   Manufacturer's Name: _____

Note that although the labels shown in Figures 6-8 and 6-9 identify the same medication, nitroglycerin, there are important differences in these two preparations. Compare the two with respect to:

	Nitroglycerin Tablets	Nitro-Bid Plateau Caps
Route		
Dosage Strength		
Form		
Manufacturer		

(*Note:* See Appendix C for answer keys.)

Practice: Reading Labels and Clinical Calculations Involving Medications Administered by the Oral Route (po)

1. **Order:** Prednisone 20 mg po
   Label: Figure 6-10
   How many tablets should be administered? _____

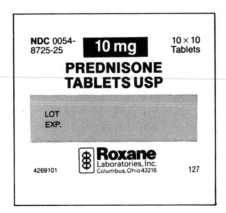

Figure 6-10   *(Courtesy Roxane Laboratories, Inc.)*

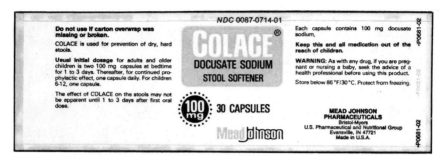

Figure 6-11 *(Courtesy Mead Johnson Pharmaceuticals)*

2. **Order:** Docusate Sodium 100 mg po
   Label: Figure 6-11
   How many capsules should be administered? _____

3. **Order:** Hydroxyzine Pamoate 60 mg po
   Label: Figure 6-12
   How many ml should be administered? _____

4. **Order:** Nilstat Suspension 1 tsp po
   Label: Figure 6-13. What is the generic name? _____
   How many units should be administered? _____

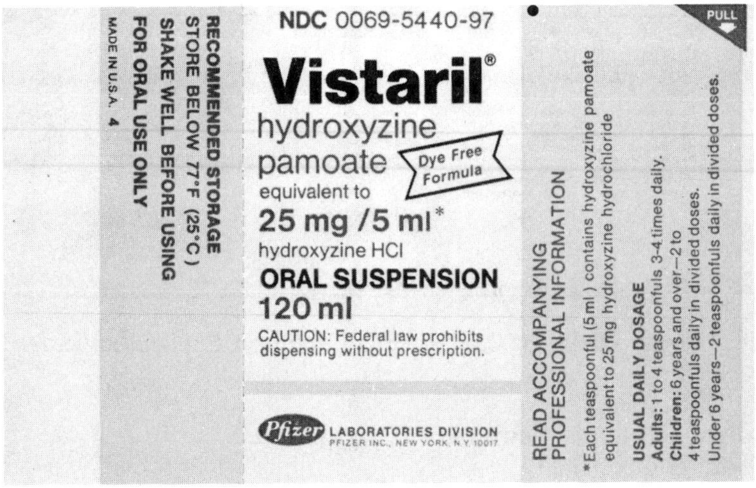

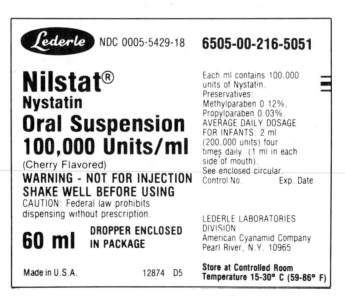

Figure 6-12   *(Courtesy Pfizer Laboratories Division, Pfizer Inc.)*

Figure 6-13   *(Courtesy Lederle Laboratories)*

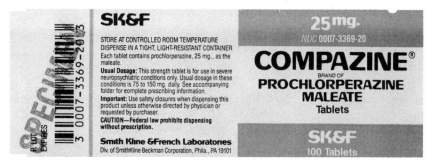

Figure 6-14   *(Courtesy Smith Kline & French Laboratories, a Division of Smith-Kline Beckman Corporation)*

5. **Order:** Compazine 50 mg po
   Label: Figure 6-14. What is the generic name? _____
   How many tablets should be administered? _____

(*Note:* See Appendix C for answer key.)

Calculations Based on Body Weight

Medications may be prescribed according to a designated amount of drug per kilogram or pound of body weight. Specific amounts of drug per unit of body weight are recommended by the drug manufacturer, and this information can be found in the product insert or in a drug reference publication. Medication orders may be written in amounts for individual doses or for total daily (24 hr) dosage, in which case the total calculated dosage must be divided by the specified number of doses to be given.

Because the amount of medication to be given is determined by the weight of the person, this weight and the calculated dosage can be considered an equivalent relationship. Our goal is to convert a particular quantity of weight to a corresponding quantity of medication. Therefore, the starting factor is in *lb* or *kg* and the answer label is in whatever units the medication is dispensed (e.g., *ml, mg, tab,* etc.).

Examples:

1. **Order:** Thiabendazole Suspension 25 mg/kg/24 hr po to an adult weighing 148 lb

Label: Thiabendazole Suspension 500 mg/5 ml
How many ml should be administered?

Starting Factor   Answer Label
    148 lb   ml

Equivalents: 2.2 lb = 1 kg, 25 mg = 1 kg, 500 mg = 5 ml

Conversion Equation: $148 \text{ lb} \times \dfrac{1 \text{ kg}}{2.2 \text{ lb}} \times \dfrac{25 \text{ mg}}{1 \text{ kg}} = \dfrac{5 \text{ ml}}{500 \text{ mg}} = 16.8 \text{ ml}$

In the first example, the total calculated dosage is administered in one dose. If the order specifies administering the medication in divided doses, it is necessary to divide the total calculated dosage by the number of doses prescribed so that the correct amount per dose will be administered.

2. **Order:** Chloromycetin 50 mg/kg/day in four divided doses po to an adult weighing 80 kg

   Label: Chloromycetin (chloramphenicol) 250 mg/cap
   How many capsules should be administered *per dose?*

   Starting Factor   Answer Label
       80 kg   cap

   Equivalents: 50 mg = 1 kg, 1 cap = 250 mg

   Conversion Equation: $80 \text{ kg} \times \dfrac{50 \text{ mg}}{1 \text{ kg}} \times \dfrac{1 \text{ cap}}{250 \text{ mg}} = \dfrac{16 \text{ cap}}{4 \text{ doses}} = 4 \text{ cap/dose}$

3. **Order:** Ancobon 50 mg/kg/day in four divided doses po to an adult weighing 135 lb

   Label: Ancobon (flucytosine) 250 mg/cap
   How many capsules should be administered *per dose?*

   Starting Factor   Answer Label
       135 lb   cap

   Equivalents: 1 kg = 2.2 lb, 50 mg = 1 kg, 1 cap = 250 mg
   Conversion Equation:

   $$135 \text{ lb} \times \dfrac{1 \text{ kg}}{2.2 \text{ lb}} \times \dfrac{50 \text{ mg}}{1 \text{ kg}} \times \dfrac{1 \text{ cap}}{250 \text{ mg}} = \dfrac{12.2 \text{ cap}}{4 \text{ doses}} = 3 \text{ cap/dose}$$

> **Remember: It is critically important to perform this final step in computations based on body weight. Consistency in this regard helps avoid errors when medication is to be given in divided doses. If this step is omitted, it is easy to forget to divide the total daily dose into the prescribed number of doses, thus greatly increasing the risk of administering an overdosage.**

Although all of the examples in this unit and Units 8 and 10 illustrate calculations of *adult* dosages based on body weight, the same method is used to calculate *pediatric* dosages also based on body weight.

Practice: Oral Dosage Based on Body Weight

1. **Order:** Ethambutol 15 mg/kg/24 hr po to an adult weighing 130 lb
   Label: Ethambutol 400 mg/tab
   How many tablets should be administered per dose?

2. **Order:** Flucytosine 50 mg/kg/day po in four divided doses to an adult
           weighing 69.4 kg
   Label: Flucytosine 250 mg/cap
   How many capsules should be administered per dose?

3. **Order:** Antiminth Oral Suspension 11 mg/kg po, one dose only, to an
           adult weighing 146 lb
   Label: Antiminth (pyrantel pamoate) Oral Suspension 50 mg/ml
   How many ml should be administered?

4. **Order:** Myambutal 25 mg/kg/24 hr po to an adult weighing 72.7 kg
   Label: Myambutal (ethambutol HCl) 400 mg/tab (scored)
   How many tablets should be administered per dose?

5. **Order:** Isoniazid Tablets 5 mg/kg po in two divided doses to an adult
   weighing 175 lb
   Label: Isoniazid Tablets 100 mg/tab
   How many tablets should be administered per dose?

Practice: Clinical Calculations Involving Medications Administered by the Oral Route (po).

A. Use the label factor method and calculate the correct amount to be
   administered per dose.

1. The physician ordered Celestone 1.8 mg po. The drug container
   label states: Celestone (beta-methasone) 0.6 mg/tablet. How
   many tablets should the patient receive?

2. The physician ordered Erythromycin 150 mg po. The label states:
   Erythromycin 0.75 Gm/fluid ounce. How many milliliters should
   be administered?

3. Aspirin gr 10 po is ordered for the patient. The strength on
   hand is Aspirin 0.3 Gm/tablet. How many tablets should be
   administered?

4. Digoxin Elixir Pediatric 0.12 mg is ordered po. The drug container label states: Digoxin 0.05 mg/ml. How many milliliters should the patient receive?

5. The physician ordered Coumadin gr ⅙ po. How many tablets should the patient receive if the label states: Coumadin (warfarin sodium) 5 mg/tablet?

6. Prolixin 0.125 mg is ordered po. The strength on hand is Prolixin (fluphenazine) 0.25 mg/tablet (scored). How many tablets should be administered?

7. The patient is to receive Penicillin G 400,000 Units po. The drug label states: Penicillin G 800,000 Units/tablet (scored). How many tablets should be administered?

8. Keflex 1 Gm po is ordered. The strength on hand is Keflex (cephalexin) 250 mg/capsule. How many capsules should the nurse administer?

9. The physician ordered Chloral Hydrate gr xv po hs. The label states: Chloral Hydrate 500 mg/dram. How many ʒ should the patient receive?

10. Nembutal Elixir 60 mg po is ordered. The label states: Nembutal (pentobarbital) Elixir 20 mg/5 ml. How many milliliters should the patient receive?

11. **Order:** Slo-Phylin 75 mg po
    Label: Slo-Phylin (theophylline) 80 mg/15 ml
    How many ml should be administered?

12. **Order:** Aminophylline 300 mg po
    Label: Aminophylline 0.1 Gm/tab
    How many tablets should the patient receive?

13. **Order:** Azulfidine 1.5 Gm po
    Label: Azulfidine (sulfasalazine) 500 mg/tab
    How many tablets should be administered?

14. **Order:** Chloromycetin 0.5 Gm po
    Label: Chloromycetin (chloramphenicol) capsule 250 mg
    How many capsules should the patient receive?

15. **Order:** Feosol Elixir 300 mg po
    Label: Feosol (ferrous sulfate) Elixir 220 mg/5 ml
    How many milliliters should be administered?

16. **Order:** Terramycin 500 mg po
    Label: Terramycin (tetracycline HCl) 50 mg/ml
    How many milliliters should be administered?

17. **Order:** Haldol 1.5 mg po
    Label: Haldol (haloperidol) 0.5 mg/tab
    How many tablets should be administered?

18. **Order:** Sulfisoxazole 0.25 Gm po
    Label: Sulfisoxazole 500 mg/tab (scored)
    How many tablets should be administered?

19. **Order:** Aldomet 250 mg po
    Label: Aldomet (methyldopa) 1 Gm/tab (scored in quarters)
    How many tablets should be administered?

20. **Order:** Vibramycin 100 mg po
    Label: Vibramycin (doxycycline) 50 mg/cap
    How many capsules should be administered?

B. Calculate the correct amount per dose.
   21. **Order:** KCl 15 mEq po
       Label: KCl (potassium chloride) 5 mEq/tab

22. **Order:** Tylenol Elixir 60 mg po
    Label: Tylenol (acetaminophen) Elixir 120 mg/5 ml

23. **Order:** Nembutal Sodium gr iss po
    Label: Nembutal Sodium (pentobarbital) 100 mg/cap

24. **Order:** Benadryl Elixir 20 mg po
    Label: Benadryl (diphenhydramine HCl) Elixir 2.5 mg/ml

25. **Order:** Phenergan 0.05 Gm po
    Label: Phenergan (promethazine HCl) 12.5 mg/tab

26. **Order:** Prolixin 1 mg po
    Label: Prolixin (fluphenazine) 2 mg/tab (scored)

27. **Order:** Gantrisin 750 mg po
    Label: Gantrisin (sulfisoxazole) 0.5 Gm/tab (scored)

28. **Order:** Compazine Syrup 2.5 mg po
    Label: Compazine (prochlorperazine) Syrup 5 mg/5 ml

29. **Order:** Lanoxin 0.125 mg po
    Label: Lanoxin (digoxin) 0.25 mg/tab (scored)

30. **Order:** Codeine Sulfate gr ¼ po
    Label: Codeine Sulfate 15 mg/tab

31. **Order:** Phenobarbital 15 mg po
    Label: Phenobarbital tablets gr ¼

32. **Order:** Seconal Sodium gr i$\overline{ss}$ po
    Label: Seconal Sodium (secobarbital) 50 mg/cap

33. **Order:** Ascorbic Acid 0.1 Gm po
    Label: Ascorbic Acid 50 mg/tab

34. **Order:** Dilantin Elixir 100 mg po
    Label: Dilantin (phenytoin sodium) Elixir 125 mg/5 ml

35. **Order:** Dilaudid Cough Syrup 3 mg po
    Label: Dilaudid (dilaudid with quaifenesin) Cough Syrup
    1 mg/5 ml
    (Give _____ tsp)

36. **Order:** Mysoline Suspension 125 mg po
    Label: Mysoline (primidone) Suspension 250 mg/5 ml

37. **Order:** Aldomet Oral Suspension 400 mg po
    Label: Aldomet (methyldopa) Oral Suspension 250 mg/5 ml

38. **Order:** Mylicon 80 mg po
    Label: Mylicon (simethicone) 40 mg/0.6 ml

39. **Order:** Mycostatin 1,000,000 U po
    Label: Mycostatin (nystatin) 500,000 U/tab

40. **Order:** Cleocin 150 mg po
    Label: Cleocin (clindamycin) 75 mg/cap

41. **Order:** Synthroid 0.2 mg po
    Label: Synthroid (levothyroxine sodium) 200 mcg/tab

42. **Order:** Sulfadiazine 1.5 Gm po
    Label: Sulfadiazine 500 mg/tab

43. **Order:** Equanil 0.2 Gm po
    Label: Equanil (meprobamate) 400 mg/tab (scored)

44. **Order:** Phenergan Syrup 25 mg po
    Label: Phenergan (promethazine HCl) Syrup 6.25 mg/5 ml

45. **Order:** Neg Gram Suspension 1 Gm po
    Label: Neg Gram (nalidixic acid) Suspension 250 mg/5 ml

46. **Order:** Minetezol Suspension 25 mg/kg/dose po to an adult
    weighing 110 lb
    Label: Minetezol (thiabendazole) Suspension 500 mg/5 ml
    How many ml should be administered per dose?

47. **Order:** Myambutol 25 mg/kg/day to an adult weighing 137 lb
    Label: Myambutol (ethambutol HCl) 400 mcg/tab
    How many tablets should be administered per dose?

48. **Order:** Nydrazid 5 mg/kg in two divided doses to an adult
    weighing 115 lb
    Label: Nydrazid (nystatin) 100 mg/tab
    How many tablets should be administered per dose?

49. **Order:** Trimethoprim 20 mg/kg/24 hr po in four divided doses
     to an adult weighing 70 kg
    Label: Trimethoprim 160 mg/tab
    How many tablets should be administered per dose?

50. **Order:** Sulfamethoxole 100 mg/kg/24 hr po in four divided
     doses to an adult weighing 154 lb
    Label: Sulfamethoxole 800 mg/tab
    How many tablets should be administered per dose?

(*Note:* See Appendix C for answer key.)

Administration of Oral Medications

···

Objectives

Upon completion of this unit of study you should be able to:
- *Interpret and follow a medication order for the purpose of administering oral medications.*
- *List the standard abbreviations used in prescribing and administering medications.*
- *Identify various routes for administering medications.*
- *List the general rules for safe administration of oral medications: pouring, administering, and recording.*
- *Identify performance criteria related to administering oral medications.*
- *Perform a simulated administration of oral medications.*

Medication Order

A physician's order is required for medications administered by nurses. This must be a written order signed by the physician. Hospital policies and procedures for medication orders vary, but in most agencies these orders are written on a special form that is a part of the patient's permanent record. The nurse should be sure that a written and signed order exists for any medication given. The only exception to this rule would be under special circumstances, such as emergencies, where a physician may give a verbal order, either directly or by phone. The registered nurse may write the order; the physician must later sign it.

The physician's order (Figure 7-1) consists of the:

1. Patient's name
2. Date and time order is written·
3. Name and dosage of medication (*Note:* Name may be written as generic or brand (trade) and dosage may be written in metric, apothecaries, or household systems.)
4. Route of administration
5. Time and frequency of administration
6. Physician's signature

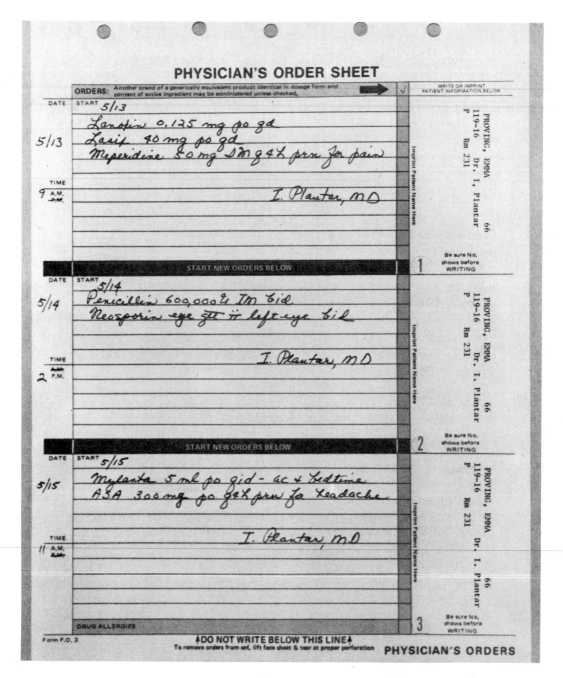

Figure 7-1   *(Courtesy of John C. Moore Corporation)*

Abbreviations

Many abbreviations are used in prescribing and administering medications. Most of these have been standardized through common usage; however, occasionally, more than one form is acceptable. To facilitate memorization, commonly used abbreviations have been divided into those dealing with amount or dosage, preparations, routes and times of administration, and any special instructions. Some, which have been introduced in earlier units, are repeated here.

Nurses should know the abbreviations listed in Tables 7-1, 7-2, 7-3, 7-4, and 7-5.

Table 7-1. AMOUNT/DOSAGE

ABBREVIATION	LATIN DERIVATION	ENGLISH
C	conguis	gallon
cc		cubic centimeter
Gm	gramma	gram
gr	granum	grain
gtt	gutta	drop
lb	libra	pound
m	minimum	minim
ml		milliliter
no	numerus	number
pt	octarius	pint
qs	quantum sifficit	quantity sufficient
ss	semis	one half
℥	dracama	dram
℥	uncia	ounce

Table 7-2. PREPARATIONS

ABBREVIATION	LATIN DERIVATION	ENGLISH
cap	capsula	capsule
elix	elixir	elixir
EC		enteric coated
ext	extractum	extract
fl	fluidus	fluid
pil	pilula	pill
sol	solutio	solution
supp	suppositorium	suppository
susp		suspension
syr	syrupus	syrup
tab	tabella	tablet
tr	tincture	tincture
ung	unguentum	ointment

Table 7-3. ROUTES

ABBREVIATION	LATIN DERIVATION	ENGLISH
ID		intradermal
IM		intramuscular
IV		intravenous
OD	oculus dexter	right eye
OS	oculus sinister	left eye
OU	oculo utro	both eyes
AD	auricula dexter	right ear
AS	auricula sinister	left ear
AU	auriculi utro	both ears
po (o)	per os	by mouth
sc	sub cutis	subcutaneous
sl	sub lingual	sublingual

Table 7-4. TIMES

ABBREVIATION	LATIN DERIVATION	ENGLISH
ā	ante	before
ac	ante cibum	before meals
am	ante meridian	before noon
bid	bis in die	*twice a day
h	hora	hour
hs	hora somni	hour of sleep or at bedtime
noct	noctis	night
o	omnis	every
od	omni die	every day
oh	omni hora	every hour
p	post	after
pc	post cibum	after meals
pm	post meridian	after noon
prn	pro re nata	whenever necessary
q	quaque	every
qd	quaque die	every day
qh (q3h, etc.)	quaque hora	*every hour (every 3 hours, etc.)
qid	quater in die	*four times a day
qod		every other day
sos	si opus sit	if necessary (one dose only)
tid	ter in die	three times a day

Note: Medications ordered q2h, q3h, q4h, etc., are given "around the clock" (i.e., throughout a 24-hour period). It is important not to confuse these abbreviations with bid, which means to administer twice a day (not every 2 hours), and qid, which means to administer 4 times a day (not every 4 hours).

Table 7-5. SPECIAL INSTRUCTIONS

ABBREVIATION	LATIN DERIVATION	ENGLISH
aa	ana (Gr.)	of each
ad lib	ad libitum	as desired
c̄	cum	with
dil	dilutus	dilute
per	per	through or by
Rx	recipe	take (or prescription)
s̄	sine	without
stat	statim	immediately

Self-Quiz—Abbreviations

A. Match abbreviations or symbols with correct meaning.

_____ 1. gtt

_____ 2. ʒ

_____ 3. sos

_____ 4. qh

_____ 5. ad lib

_____ 6. bid

_____ 7. ext

_____ 8. c̄

_____ 9. stat

_____ 10. q

A. as desired
B. dram
C. drop
D. every
E. every hour
F. extract
G. fluid
H. immediately
I. one dose only
J. ounce
K. three times a day
L. twice a day
M. whenever necessary
N. with

B. Write the term.

1. ac = _____

2. cap = _____

3. Gm = _____

4. pc = _____

5. q3h = _____

6. s̄ = _____

7. elix = _____

8. prn = _____

9. ss = _____

10. ml = _____

C. Identify the route.

1. IM = _____

2. IV = _____

3. sc = _____

4. OS = _____

5. OD = _____   8. sl = _____
6. OU = _____   9. ID = _____
7. po = _____

(*Note:* See appendix C for answer key.)

Routes for Administering Medications

The common routes by which medications are administered are:

- mouth—po
- swish and swallow—S & S
- injection (parenteral)
  —subcutaneous—sc
  —intramuscular—IM
  —intradermal—ID
  —intravenous—IV
  —intrathecal (into the spinal canal) ⎫
  —intracardial (into the heart)   ⎬ Less common parenteral routes
  —intra-articular (into a joint)   ⎭
- inhalation—respiratory tract
- topical—placing on skin, mucous membrane, or in body cavity
  —sublingual (under the tongue)
  —instillation (dropping liquid into a cavity: eye drops)
  —inunction (rubbing ointment on skin)
  —irrigation (into a wound or body cavity)
  —suppository (vaginal, rectal, urethral)
  —patch (applied to the skin, with medication absorbed through the skin)

The Medication Kardex (Medex)

Safe nursing practice requires the use of some type of medication administration record (MAR) or guide to which the nurse can refer when administering medications. Usually this is in the form of a special Kardex, sometimes called a Medex, on which all medication orders for individual patients are reproduced on separate cards or pages. Figure 7-2 is a sample Kardex.

Note that the patient's name and room number appear on the card, along with all pertinent information relating to the order: drug, dose, route, date, and time of administration. As a rule, space for recording each dose given also appears on the card. If pertinent, start and stop dates and special instructions or precautions are included. The presence or absence of allergies should be noted by listing any substance to which the patient is allergic or by using some notation such as NKA (no known

COMMUNITY HOSPITAL

NURSE'S SIGNATURE	INIT.	NURSE'S SIGNATURE	INIT.	NURSE'S SIGNATURE	INIT.
Marilyn Lust RN	ml				
A Donald Insley R.N.	ADI				
Rosemary Fischer RN	RF				
M Kathleen Wecker RN	MKW				
Joan Carretta RN	JC				
Teresa Bericat SN	TB				

RA-Right Arm RB-Right Buttocks RL-Right Leg LA-Left Arm LB-Left Buttocks LL-Left Leg

ROUTINE MEDICATION ORDERS

ORD DATE	EXP DATE	Medication Frequency	Dosage Route	Shift	DATE HOUR	5/13 INIT.	6/14 INIT.	5/15 INIT.	5/16 INIT.	5/17 INIT.	5/18 INIT.	5/19 INIT.
5/13		LANOXIN	0.125mg	11-7								
		qd	po	7-3	9	ml	ml	ADI	TB			
				3-11		P74	P72	P77	P68			
5/13		LASIX	40mg	11-7								
		qd	po	7-3	9	ml	ml	ADI	TB			
				3-11								
5/14		PENICILLIN G	600000U	11-7		X						
		bid	IM	7-3	9	X	ml/LL	ADI/LB	TB/LL			
				3-11	9	X	RF/LA	RF/RB	JC/RL			
5/14		NEOSPORIN eye gtt ii	OS	11-7		X						
		bid		7-3	10	X	ml	ADI	TB			
				3-11	6	X	RF	RF	JC			
5/15		MYLANTA	5ml	11-7		X	X					
		qid (AC + HS)	po	7-3	7^{30}-11^{30}	X	X	ADI / ADI	TB / TB			
				3-11	4^{30}-9	X	X	RF / RF	JC / JC			
				11-7								
				7-3								
				3-11								

PRN MEDICATIONS

DOCUMENT PRN INJECTION SITE IN NURSE'S NOTES

ORD DATE	EXP DATE	Medication Frequency	Dosage Route	Doses Given			
5/13	5/15	Meperidine	50mg	Date	5/13	5/14	5/15
		IM q4h PRN		Time	12^{30}	9^{P}	2^{30}
		for pain		INIT	ml	RF	mKW
5/15		ASA 300mg po		Date	5/15	5/16	
		q3h PRN FOR HEADACHE		Time	4:^{00}a	12^{N}	
				INIT	ADI.	mKW	
				Date			
				Time			
				INIT			
				Date			
				Time			
				INIT			

Room No.:	Name:	Hosp. No.:	Age:	Physician:
231	EMMA PROVING	119-16	66	I PLANTAR, M.D

Allergies: NKA

Figure 7-2 Kardex—record of administration of medications

allergies). As the medication Kardex is filled up or discontinued, it becomes part of the patient's permanent record.

A nurse should never give a medication without referring to this reproduction of the medication order or, if there is any question, to the original order in the patient's medical record. It is essential that the Medex be up to date and that any delayed or temporarily omitted medication (e.g., patient fasting for test or on call for surgery, etc.) be identified appropriately so it is not administered inadvertently.

Recording Medications

All medications given must be recorded immediately on the patient's Medex or medical record, according to the policy of the institution. Only the nurse who administered the medications should sign for them. Usually initials are used for recording, with a place for the full signature somewhere on the sheet or card. There is usually some method for indicating that a medication has been omitted. Whenever this occurs, the reason for the omission should be recorded in the nurse's notes. All narcotics and other controlled drugs must be accounted for on a special record (e.g., narcotic log), again according to the policy of the institution. In some institutions, medication documentation may be computerized.

The importance of accurate recording of medications cannot be overemphasized. Refer to Figure 7-2 for an example of such documentation.

Drug Distribution System

The physician may order a drug by either its generic name or a brand name. This is the name that will be transcribed to the Medex. Because of the price differences that may exist between generic and brand name products, many hospital pharmacies are currently dispensing generic drugs, insofar as possible. Therefore, the nurse frequently may find a drug labeled by the generic name, rather than the name under which it was ordered. It is essential to verify that the correct drug is being given; a comparison handbook, the *Physician's Desk Reference,* a pharmacist, or some other source should be available for this purpose. The importance of this verification cannot be overemphasized.

The unit dose system is being used more frequently as a method of dispensing drugs. With this method, premeasured drugs are packaged individually and usually are not opened until the time of administration. This method reduces the chance of error, as well as the time spent in preparing and pouring medications. In many instances, the necessity for computation is eliminated, because the drug is dispensed in the same dosage strength as the ordered dose. The nurse still must verify that the correct medication and dose are being administered. Some agencies still may be dispensing medications from labeled containers, rather than unit doses, in which case the nurse has greater responsibility for obtaining and verifying the correct dose.

Accountability

The nurse is accountable for safe practice in administering medications. This includes questioning and verifying any physician's order that is outside the normal dosage range, as recommended by the drug manufacturer's product insert or a drug reference manual. The nurse should question any medication order that might be contraindicated due to the patient's current condition or that may appear to be having an adverse effect. Moreover, the nurse must be alert for drug allergies, incompatibilities, or interactions, and must have knowledge of appropriate nursing implications and interventions relative to the drugs being administered.

General Rules for Administration of Medications

In the administration of medications, regardless of the route used, the nurse should do the following:

1. Always have a physician's order for medications administered.
2. Wash hands before pouring any medication.
3. Concentrate entirely on preparing and administering medications. Do not allow distractions to interfere with this procedure.
4. Refer to a Medex (Medication Kardex) for every medication administered, one that corresponds exactly with the physician's order.
5. Check for any known drug allergies the patient might have.
6. If the unit dose system is employed, check the prepackaged unit label against the Medex when obtaining any prepackaged medications from patient's storage area.
7. If a stock or patient supply system is employed, read the label of the medication three times and check with the Medex:
   a. when obtaining the container
   b. just before pouring the medication
   c. immediately after pouring the dose
8. Obtain medications only from legibly labeled containers.
9. Check to be sure the medication is not outdated or has an abnormal appearance.
10. Check the Medex or prn sheet for the time of the most recent administration of a prn medication.
11. Record controlled drugs on the appropriate control sheet when the medication is removed from a locked cupboard.
12. Do not administer medications that have been poured or prepared by another person. **Exception:** If the unit dose system is employed, individual doses will have been dispensed by the pharmacist. The

nurse must still verify that the correct medication and dose are administered.

13. Ascertain pertinent information about medications being administered: action, results expected, untoward effects, usual dose, and/or special nursing considerations.

14. Keep the medication cart or tray within sight at all times.

15. Before administering the medication, identify the patient by asking or stating the patient's name, *examining the wristband,* and comparing the information on the wristband to the medication administration guide (Medex, medication sheet, etc.).

16. If the patient questions or expresses concern about a medication, withhold the medication long enough to re-check the order, the medication, and the dose.

17. If the patient refuses a medication, attempt to ascertain the reason and report and record this information appropriately.

18. Before administering a medication, perform any pertinent assessment relative to the medication; check pulse, blood pressure, respiration, reflexes, pupillary size, etc.

19. Remain with the patient until the medication is taken. Never leave the medication at the patient's bedside without an order from the physician.

20. Maintain an aseptic (clean) technique throughout the procedure.

21. Record the medication immediately after administering it. Observe the patient for desired or undesired effects and report and/or document any pertinent information.

22. Remember the SIX RIGHTS. Administer:
    - the right medication.
    - to the right patient.
    - at the right time.
    - in the right amount.
    - by the right route.
    - with the right documentation.

Administering Oral Medications

In administration of oral medications, it is important to keep in mind the following:

- Check to determine if:
    —the dose should be withheld (NPO, nausea, etc.).
    —a previously delayed dose that is given once daily may now be administered (test completed, etc.).

—a previously delayed dose that is given several times a day may now be administered according to daily schedule.

■ When dispensing prepackaged doses, open the packets at bedside just prior to administration.

■ When dispensing pills, tablets, or capsules that are not wrapped, use the cap of the container to transfer the medication into the medicine cup. If possible, the fingers should not come into contact with the drugs.

■ If tablets are scored, they may be broken into halves or quarters if necessary. In many agencies, this is done in the pharmacy prior to dispensing.

■ If several tablets, pills, or capsules are to be given at one time, they may be poured into the same cup, with the exception of any medications that require assessment prior to administration (e.g., checking pulse, BP, or reflex). These should be poured separately as a reminder or because they may have to be omitted.

■ Use a medicine dropper to measure medications ordered in drops.

■ In pouring liquid medications, place the thumbnail on the medicine glass marking the correct dose and pour at eye level or with the glass on a flat surface. (Palm label to pour and wipe off lip of bottle, as necessary.)

■ The measure of liquid medicine is read at the lowest point of the meniscus.

■ Liquid medications may or may not need to be diluted with water or another liquid. Check specific instructions.

■ Crush, dissolve, and/or mix medications with small amount of food or liquid as necessary. **Exceptions:** capsules, enteric-coated tablets, or time-release drugs.

■ Assist patients to take their medications:
   —elevate head of bed.
   —assess swallowing ability.
   —have water available at bedside.
   —if several tablets are to be taken, offer them one at a time.
   —give sips of water after each tablet to increase fluid intake.
   —make sure patient has swallowed all medications.
   —medications administered sublingually, chewables, or medications that should not be followed by water should be given last.

■ Record amount of liquid given on Fluid Balance Sheet, if indicated.

The learner may find the following checklist a helpful guide for the administration of oral medications.

Performance Criteria: Administration of Oral Medications

	S	U	Comments
A. Prior to administration 1. Obtains Medication Medex to confirm medication order regarding dose, route, and time of administration			
2. Checks for any known allergies			
3. Washes hands			
B. Administration of tablets or capsules 1. Obtains correct medication			
2. Checks the label against the Medex			
3. a. Pours the correct dose into bottle cap and then into cup; recaps medicine bottle and re-checks label against the Medex **OR** b. Selects prepackaged unit dose, checks label against Medex, then places wrapped medication in cup			
4. If controlled drugs are dispensed, maintains security of storage area and documents (records) in appropriate manner			
5. Confirms patient's identity by asking or stating patient's name and checking wristband against Medex/med sheet			
6. If necessary, assesses pulse, blood pressure, etc. as appropriate for medication being administered			
7. Elevates head, as necessary			

Continued on next page

Performance Criteria: Administration of Oral Medications (Cont.)

	S	U	Comments
8. Hands the medicine cup to the patient or taps the medicine into the patient's hand or directly into the patient's mouth			
9. Gives water or juice to assist in swallowing medication			
10. For sublingual medication, instructs patient to place tablet under tongue and hold in place until it is absorbed			
11. For buccal medication, instructs patient to place tablet between cheek and teeth, close mouth, and hold tablet against cheek until absorbed			
C. Administration of liquid medications 1. Obtains correct medication and checks the label against the Medex			
2. Shakes well, if in suspension			
3. Uncaps the bottle and places the cap open side up on a clean surface			
4. Holds the medicine cup at eye level			
5. Places thumbnail on the correct marking on medicine cup			
6. Pours correct amount of medication, measuring at lowest point of meniscus			
7. Re-checks the poured dosage by setting cup on level surface and reading meniscus at eye level			
8. Re-checks the label against the Medex			

Continued on next page

Performance Criteria: Administration of Oral Medications (Cont.)

	S	U	Comments
9. Wipes the bottle top with a damp paper towel and replaces cap			
10. Confirms patient's identity by asking or stating name and checking wristband against Medex/med sheet			
11. Elevates head, as necessary			
12. Hands medicine cup to patient or assists as needed a. Uses a straw for medications which stain the teeth (iron, hydrochloric acid, etc.)			
b. Follows medication with water, if indicated			
c. Omits water if contraindicated			
D. Administration of liquid medications via syringe 1. Obtains correct medication and checks the label against the Medex			
2. Selects correct size syringe according to desired dosage			
3. a. Pours medication into a medicine cup and withdraws the dosage into the syringe **OR** b. Withdraws the medication into the syringe via a sterile needle, then discards the needle			
4. Obtains correct dose			
5. Checks dosage in syringe making sure there are no air bubbles displacing medication			
6. Re-checks the label against the Medex			

Continued on next page

Performance Criteria: Administration of Oral Medications (Cont.)

	S	U	Comments
7. Confirms patient's identity by asking or stating the patient's name and checking wristband against Medex/med sheet			
8. Places syringe tip in side of patient's mouth and instills the medication slowly			
E. Following administration of medication 1. Remains with patient until medication is taken			
2. Records accurately on Medex and/or nursing notes			
3. Records fluids given, if indicated			
4. Provides proper after care of equipment			
F. Maintains principles of asepsis throughout the procedure			
G. Maintains principles of patient safety and comfort throughout the procedure			

S—Satisfactory   U—Unsatisfactory   Evaluator _____

Practice: Simulated Medication Administration Using Medex

The labels in Figure 7-3 represent medications found in a patient's medication storage area. Figure 7-4 is the Medex card for this patient.

1. Assume you are to administer the 9:00 A.M. oral medications. In the chart on page 89, record the quantity (ml, capsules, tablets, etc.) of each medication you would administer. In some instances no computation is necessary, because it can be determined by inspection of the label or by simple mental arithmetic. When it is necessary to calculate, *use the label factor method.*

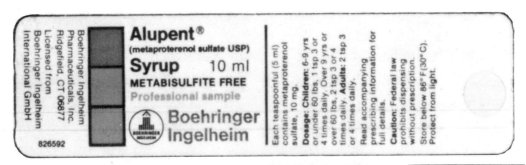

Alupent®
(metaproterenol sulfate USP)

Syrup   10 ml
METABISULFITE FREE
Professional sample

Boehringer
Ingelheim

Boehringer Ingelheim
Pharmaceuticals, Inc.
Ridgefield, CT 06877
Licensed from
Boehringer Ingelheim
International GmbH

826592

Each teaspoonful (5 ml) contains metaproterenol sulfate, 10 mg.

Dosage: Children: 6-9 yrs or under 60 lbs, 1 tsp 3 or 4 times daily. Over 9 yrs or over 60 lbs, 2 tsp 3 or 4 times daily. Adults: 2 tsp 3 or 4 times daily.

Read accompanying prescribing information for full details.

Caution: Federal law prohibits dispensing without prescription.

Store below 86° F (30° C). Protect from light.

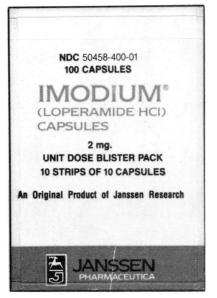

NDC 50458-400-01
100 CAPSULES

IMODIUM®
(LOPERAMIDE HCl)
CAPSULES

2 mg.
UNIT DOSE BLISTER PACK
10 STRIPS OF 10 CAPSULES

An Original Product of Janssen Research

JANSSEN
PHARMACEUTICA

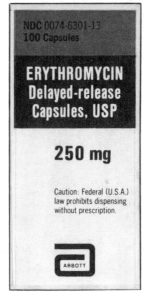

NDC 0074-6301-13
100 Capsules

ERYTHROMYCIN
Delayed-release
Capsules, USP

250 mg

Caution: Federal (U.S.A.) law prohibits dispensing without prescription.

ABBOTT

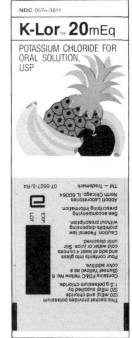

NDC 0074-3611

K-Lor™ 20mEq

POTASSIUM CHLORIDE FOR ORAL SOLUTION, USP

TM — Trademark   07-5527-5/R4

Abbott Laboratories
North Chicago, IL 60064
See accompanying
prescribing information.

Caution: Federal law
prohibits dispensing
without prescription.

Pour contents into glass
and add at least 4 ounces
cold water or juice. Stir
until dissolved.

Contains FD&C Yellow No. 6
(Sunset Yellow) as a
color additive.

This packet provides potassium
(20 mEq) and chloride
(20 mEq) supplied by
1.5 g potassium chloride.

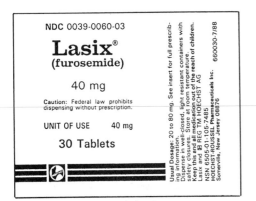

NDC 0039-0060-03

Lasix®
(furosemide)

40 mg

Caution: Federal law prohibits
dispensing without prescription.

UNIT OF USE   40 mg

30 Tablets

Usual Dosage: 20 to 80 mg. See insert for full prescrib-
ing information. Dispense in well-closed, light resistant containers with
safety closures. Store at room temperature.
Keep this and all medication out of the reach of children.
Lasix and ℞ REG TM HOECHST AG
NSN 6505-01-105-7485
HOECHST-ROUSSEL Pharmaceuticals Inc.
Somerville, New Jersey 08876

660030-7/88

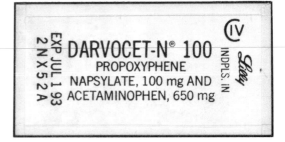

EXP JUL 1 93
2 N X 5 2 A

DARVOCET-N® 100
PROPOXYPHENE
NAPSYLATE, 100 mg AND
ACETAMINOPHEN, 650 mg

C IV
INDPLS, IN

Figure 7-3 *(Labels courtesy E. R. Squibb & Sons, Inc., Hoechst-Roussel Phar-maceuticals Inc., Boehringer Ingelheim Pharmaceuticals, Inc., Abbott Labora-tories, Janssen Pharmaceuticals Inc., Burroughs Wellcome Co., Eli Lilly & Co., Mead Johnson Pharmaceuticals, and McNeil Pharmaceutical)*

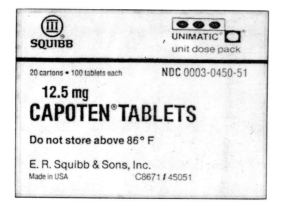

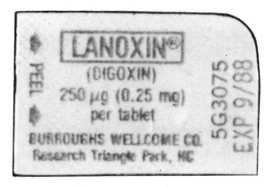

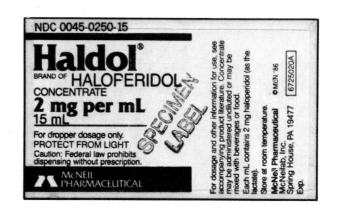

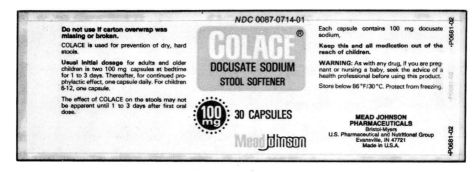

Figure 7-3 Cont.

NURSE'S SIGNATURE	INIT.	NURSE'S SIGNATURE	INIT.	NURSE'S SIGNATURE	INIT.

RA-Right Arm   RB-Right Buttocks   RL-Right Leg   LA-Left Arm   LB-Left Buttocks   LL-Left Leg

ROUTINE MEDICATION ORDERS

ORD DATE	EXP DATE	Medication Frequency	Dosage Route	Shift	DATE HOUR	→ 6/22 INIT.	6/23 INIT.	6/24 INIT.	6/25 INIT.	6/26 INIT.	6/27 INIT.	6/28 INIT.
6/22		DIGOXIN	0.25 mg	11-7	↓							
		qd	po	7-3	9							
				3-11	Pulse							
6/22		LASIX	80 mg	11-7								
		qd	po	7-3	7³⁰							
				3-11								
6/22		K LOR	20 mEq	11-7								
		tid-pc	po	7-3	9-1							
		Dissolve in 4 ℥ water or juice		3-11	6							
6/22		CAPOTEN	25 mg	11-7								
		bid-AC	po	7-3	7³⁰							
				3-11	4³⁰							
6/22		ALUPENT SYRUP	1.5 tsp	11-7								
		qid	po	7-3	9-1							
				3-11	5-9							
6/22		ERYTHROMYCIN	500 mg	11-7								
		D-R CAP	po	7-3	9							
		bid		3-11	9							
6/22		HALDOL	1.5 mg	11-7								
		tid	po	7-3	9-1							
				3-11	6							
6/22	bs	COLACE	100 mg	11-7								
		qd hs	po	7-3								
				3-11	9							

PRN MEDICATION ORDERS

ORD DATE	EXP DATE	Medication Frequency	Dosage Route		Doses Given																
6/22		IMODIUM	Cap ī	Date																	
		following each	po	Time																	
		unformed stool		INIT																	
6/22		DARVOCET N·100	ī	Date																	
		q4h prn	po	Time																	
		for pain		INIT																	

Figure 7-4   Medex card

MEDICATION	AMOUNT TO BE GIVEN

Figure 7-4 Cont.

2. The Lasix is ordered ac breakfast. How many tablets should the patient receive, and when? _____
3. The K-Lor must be dissolved in liquid prior to administration.
   ■ What liquids can be used? _____
   ■ How many ml would you record on the fluid intake record? _____
4. What is the dosage strength of the Capoten? _____
   ■ How many tablets should be administered at 7:30 A.M.? _____
5. You administered 1.5 tsp of Alupent. Using the label factor method, calculate the following:
   ■ How many ml did the patient receive? _____
   ■ How many mg did the patient receive? _____
   ■ The usual adult dose is 20 mg 3–4 times a day. Did this patient receive a safe dose? _____
6. How many ml does the Haldol bottle contain? _____
   ■ What is the total number of 1.5 mg doses available from this amount? _____
7. What is the dosage strength of the Docusate Sodium capsules? _____
   ■ How many capsules will the patient receive at bedtime? _____
8. The original medication order for Imodium was written: Give 2 capsules stat and 1 capsule following each unformed stool.
   ■ How many mg were administered stat? _____
   ■ How many mg are to be administered following each unformed stool? _____
9. If the patient is complaining of pain, what medication may be administered? _____
   ■ How often may the patient receive this medication? _____
   ■ How many tablets would be administered per dose? _____
   ■ What is the expiration date of this medication? _____

(*Note:* See Appendix C for answer key.)

Calculation of Parenteral Medications

Objectives

Upon completion of this unit of study you should be able to:

- *Identify appropriate equipment used in the administration of parenteral medications, including types of syringes and the length and gauge of needles.*
- *Demonstrate the ability to accurately read calibrations on various types of syringes.*
- *Demonstrate knowledge of the appropriate method for rounding off doses when administering parenteral medications.*
- *Identify various forms of parenteral medications.*
- *Read drug labels to obtain information about specific parenteral drugs, including reconstitution.*
- *Apply the label factor method to clinical calculations involving drugs administered by subcutaneous and intramuscular routes.*

Parenteral Medications

Medications that are administered via injection into dermal, subcutaneous, or intramuscular tissues or directly into a vein are called parenteral medications, because they are administered by routes outside the gastrointestinal tract.

Parenteral routes include:

1. Intradermal (ID)
2. Subcutaneous (sc)
3. Intramuscular (IM)
4. Intravenous (IV)
5. Intrathecal
6. Intracardial
7. Intra-articular

This unit focuses on medications administered by intradermal, subcutaneous, and intramuscular routes. Intravenous medications will be the subject of Units 10 and 11. Intrathecal, intracardial, and intra-articular injections will be excluded, because these medication routes require specialized knowledge and training and are beyond the scope of this text.

In this unit you will learn about the equipment used in administering parenteral medications, the various forms of these medications, and how to read labels and calculate dosages.

The Syringe and Needle

The Syringe

Figure 8-1 illustrates the three parts of a syringe: the barrel contains the medication and is calibrated to measure the quantity to be given; the plunger is made of clouded or colored glass or plastic and is operated to fill or empty the barrel; the lower end of the syringe terminates in a hub to which the needle is attached. It is essential that all parts of the syringe that contact the medication be kept free of contamination. This includes the needle, the outer edge of the hub, the plunger, and the inside of the barrel.

There are various types of syringes available, most of which, at present, are single-use disposable units with attached needles. The needle usually can be detached and replaced. These syringes are made of plastic and are prepackaged in sterile packets. Reusable glass syringes are available, but their use is limited due to the increasing utilization of disposable equipment.

The syringe of choice depends on the route, action, and volume of medication to be administered.

The Tuberculin Syringe   The tuberculin syringe will measure a total of 1 cc , and is calibrated in hundredths (0.01 cc) and also in minims (15–16 m/cc). This syringe is used when very small quantities of medication must be measured (i.e., less than 1 cc). It usually is prepackaged with a 5/8″ long needle, Figure 8-2.

The Insulin Syringe   The insulin syringe is calibrated in units and should be used exclusively in the administration of insulin, because it will give the most accurate measurement (see Figure 9-15).

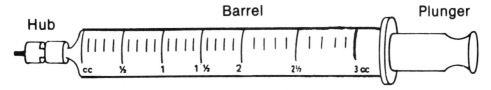

Figure 8-1   3 cc syringe

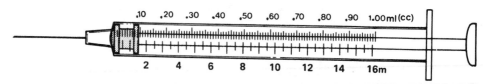

Figure 8-2   Tuberculin syringe

The 3, 5, and 10 cc Syringes   The 3 cc syringe is calibrated in tenths (0.1 cc) and also in minims. Note that on the cc side, each calibration line measures 0.1 cc.

Five and 10 cc syringes may be used when a large volume of medication is to be measured or administered. It is important to note that on the 5 and 10 cc syringes, each calibration line measures 0.2 cc, Figure 8-3.

The Needle

The choice of needle depends on the route and site of administration, the size and obesity of the patient, and the viscosity of the medication. Needles vary in length from ¼" to 3". Shorter needles (¼"–1") are used for intra-

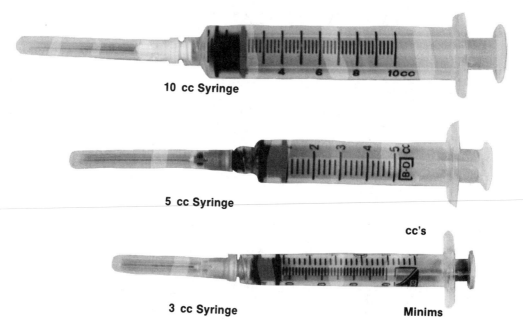

Figure 8-3   *(Courtesy Dale Green, Director, Educational Communications Center, Alfred State College)*

dermal or subcutaneous injections and/or small or thin patients; longer needles (1″–2″) are used for intramuscular injections, irritating medications, and/or larger or obese patients.

The diameter of the needle is indicated by a gauge number. Gauge number runs from 14 to 27; the larger the number, the smaller the diameter of the needle. Fine needles are used for aqueous solutions and heavier needles for suspensions and oils. The widened portion of the needle, called the hub, attaches to the syringe. The angled point, which is called the bevel, increases the sharpness of the needle. A protective cap is provided to maintain sterility. Most needles are now disposable and are destroyed after a single use, Figure 8-4.

Reading the Syringe

It is important to note that on most single-use syringes the plunger has a rubber tip that has two rings in contact with the barrel, Figure 8-5. Measurement must be made at the top ring—the one closest to the tip—in order to have an accurate dose.
Refer to Figure 8-6.

1. The 3 cc syringe contains 1.2 ml of solution.
2. The tuberculin syringe contains 0.75 ml of solution.
3. The insulin syringe contains 28 units of solution.

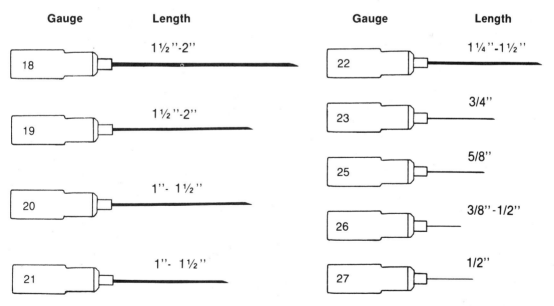

Figure 8-4

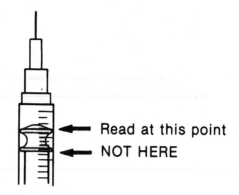

Figure 8-5

Shade in the dosage on the following syringes: Refer to Figure 8-7.

1. 14 m
2. 0.52 ml
3. 64 units

(*Note:* See Appendix C for answer key.)

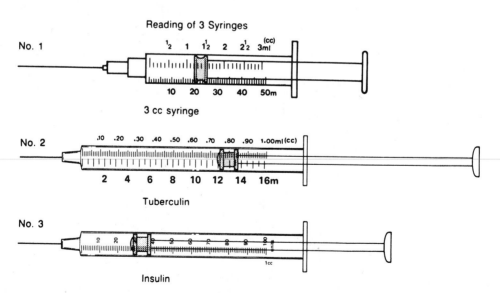

Figure 8-6

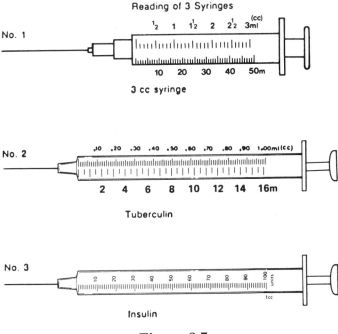

Figure 8-7

Rounding Off

Because clinical calculations will not always result in dosages of whole numbers, it is necessary to use the correct procedure for rounding off these values.

■ When the calculated dose is obtained in exact tenths of milliliters, the solution may be accurately measured in a 1, 2, or 3 milliliter syringe calibrated in tenths; refer to Figure 8-8.

1. 0.8 ml
2. 1.3 ml
3. 2.2 ml

■ When the calculated dosage does not result in exact tenths of milliliters, the decimal result is carried to hundredths and rounded in the following manner:
—If the digit in the hundredths place is less than 5, this digit is dropped.
—If the digit in the hundredths place is greater than 5, the tenths digit is increased by 1.

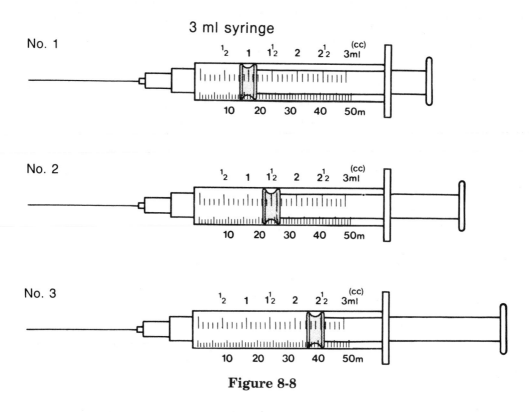

Figure 8-8

These dosages can be administered in a syringe of suitable capacity, calibrated in tenths of milliliters. For example:

1. 2.31 ml; give 2.3 ml
2. 1.87 ml; give 1.9 ml
3. 1.25 ml; give 1.3 ml

If a tuberculin syringe is used, it is possible to measure hundredths of a milliliter. Therefore, the computation should be carried to thousandths and then rounded to hundredths.

Remember: To convert ml to m, it is necessary to compare equivalent values between metric and apothecaries units of volume. One ml is equivalent to 15–16 m. Most syringes that are calibrated in both ml and m use the equivalent 16 m per ml. However, in calculating dosage conversions, it is common practice to use the equivalent 15 m per ml. In computations involving such conversions in this text, the equivalent 15 m = 1 ml will be used.

When answers are obtained in minims, decimal results should be rounded to whole numbers, because it is not possible to divide minims. **Exception:** If a tuberculin (1 ml) syringe is used, it is possible to measure 0.5 minim on the syringe; therefore, the computation should be rounded accordingly.

1. 5.7 m; give 6 m
2. 12.3 m; give 12 m
3. 22.9 m; give 23 m
4. 8.5 m; give 8.5 m (tuberculin syringe)

Parenteral Medication Forms

There are a variety of forms in which drugs for parenteral administration are available. Some come in powder form and must be reconstituted to a liquid, whereas others are in solution and are dispensed in ampules, vials, or cartridges.

Single-Dose Ampules

Most ampules have a constricted stem that facilitates snapping them open. For protection, a piece of gauze or alcohol wipe may be wrapped around the stem before it is broken (Figure 8-9). Any medication in the stem should be shaken down into the ampule before opening. A metal file or an ampule opener can be used to ensure an even break if the ampule is not pre-scored.

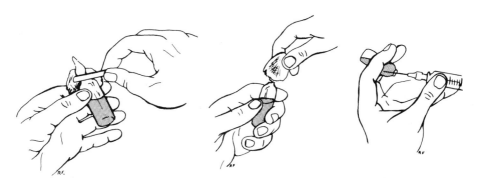

Figure 8-9 Obtaining medication from an ampule

Single- and Multiple-Dose Vials

Some drugs are dispensed in single-dose vials, whereas others are in vials containing several doses. The vial is entered through the rubber diaphragm, which should be cleansed first with an antiseptic. An amount of air comparable to the amount of drug to be withdrawn is injected. The solution can then be withdrawn easily, because fluids move from an area of greater pressure to that of a lesser pressure. It is essential that there be no air bubbles present in the measured quantity, in order to have an accurate dose (Figure 8-10).

Pre-Filled Cartridges

Some medications are dispensed in pre-measured, single-dose disposable cartridges. There may or may not be a needle attached to the cartridge. The pre-filled unit is advantageous as a time-saver and reduced risk of contamination. The unit is placed into a cartridge-holder or injector, which functions like a syringe. Excess air must be expelled from the cartridge prior to administering the medication. The cartridge-holder is reusable; the cartridge and needles are discarded after the medication is administered.

To lessen the risk of needle-stick injuries, the newer injectors are designed to eliminate the need for handling or manipulating the used cartridge or needle, Figure 8-11.

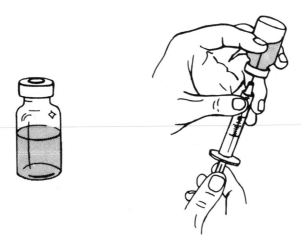

Figure 8-10   Obtaining medication from a vial

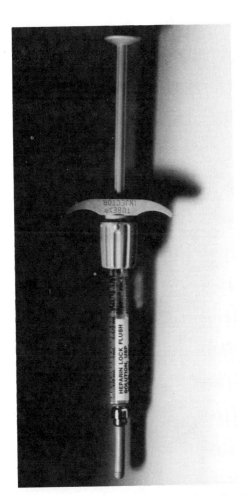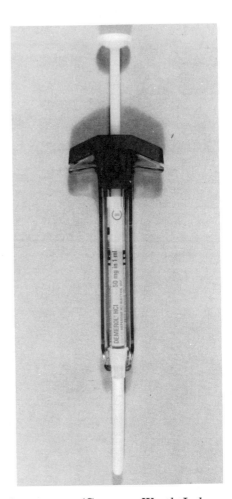

Figure 8-11 (Left) Tubex® closed injection system *(Courtesy Wyeth Laboratories)* (Right) *Carpuject*® sterile cartridge-needle unit *(Courtesy Winthrop-Breon Laboratories, Division of Sterling Drug)*

Reading Labels

The manufacturer's product insert describes, in detail, the: composition of the drug, its actions, indications and contraindications for use, precautions and adverse reactions, dosage, directions for dilution or reconstitution, if necessary, and directions for administration, Figure 8-12.

Wyeth
Omnipen®-N
(ampicillin sodium)
for **IM** or **IV** injection

A.H.F.S. Category 8:12.16

Description
Omnipen-N (ampicillin sodium) for Injection is a semisynthetic penicillin derived from the basic penicillin nucleus, 6-amino penicillanic acid.

NOTE: Omnipen-N contains 3.1 milliequivalents of sodium per gram of ampicillin as the sodium salt.

Actions
MICROBIOLOGY
In vitro studies have shown sensitivity of the following microorganisms to ampicillin:

Gram-Positive: Alpha- and beta-hemolytic streptococci, *Diplococcus pneumoniae,* staphylococci (nonpenicillinase-producing), *Bacillus anthracis,* clostridia spp., *Corynebacterium xerosis,* and most strains of enterococci.

The drug does not resist destruction by penicillinase; hence, it is not effective against penicillin-G-resistant staphylococci.

Gram-Negative: Hemophilus influenzae, Neisseria gonorrhoeae, Neisseria meningitidis, Proteus mirabilis, and many strains of Salmonella (including *Salmonella typhosa),* Shigella, and *Escherichia coli.*

Testing for Susceptibility: The invading organism should be cultured and its sensitivity demonstrated as a guide to therapy. If the Kirby-Bauer method of disc sensitivity is used, a 10-mcg ampicillin disc should be used to determine the relative *in vitro* susceptibility.

HUMAN PHARMACOLOGY
Ampicillin is stable in the presence of gastric acid and is well-absorbed from the gastrointestinal tract. It diffuses readily into most body tissues and fluids. However, penetration into the cerebrospinal fluid and brain occurs only with meningeal inflammation. Ampicillin is excreted largely unchanged in the urine. Its excretion can be delayed by concurrent administration of probenecid.

Ampicillin is the least serum-bound of all the penicillins, averaging 20% compared to 60-90% for other penicillins.

Blood serum levels obtained on IM injection are proportionate to the dose administered. Levels of approximately 40 mcg/ml per 1-gram IM dose are attained at one-half hour. Higher levels are attainable with IV injection, depending on the dose and rate of administration.

Indications
Ampicillin is indicated primarily in the treatment of infections caused by susceptible strains of the following microorganisms: Shigella, Salmonella (including *S. typhosa),* E. coli, *H. influenzae, P. mirabilis, N. gonorrhoeae,* and enterococci. It is also indicated in the treatment of meningitis due to *N. meningitidis.* Since it is effective against the commonest pathogens causing meningitis, it may be used intravenously as initial therapy before the results of bacteriology are available. Ampicillin is also indicated in certain infections caused by susceptible gram-positive organisms: penicillin-G-sensitive staphylococci, streptococci, and pneumococci. Bacteriologic studies to determine the causative organisms and their sensitivity to ampicillin should be performed. Therapy may be instituted prior to the results of culture and sensitivity testing.

It is advisable to reserve the parenteral form of this drug for moderately severe and severe infections and for patients who are unable to take the oral forms (capsules, oral suspension, or pediatric drops). A change to oral Omnipen (ampicillin) may be made as soon as appropriate.

Contraindications
Ampicillin is contraindicated in patients with a history of a hypersensitivity reaction to the penicillins.

Warnings
Serious and occasionally fatal hypersensitivity (anaphylactoid) reactions have been reported in patients on penicillin therapy. Although anaphylaxis is more frequent following parenteral therapy, it has occurred in patients on oral penicillins. These reactions are more apt to occur in individuals with a history of sensitivity to multiple allergens.

There have been reports of individuals with a history of penicillin hypersensitivity who experienced severe reactions when treated with cephalosporins. Before therapy with any penicillin, careful inquiry should be made concerning previous hypersensitivity reactions to penicillins, cephalosporins, or other allergens. If an allergic reaction occurs, appropriate therapy should be instituted and discontinuation of ampicillin therapy considered. **Serious anaphylactoid reactions require immediate emergency treatment with epinephrine. Oxygen, intra-**venous steroids, and airway management, including intubation, should be administered as indicated.

USAGE IN PREGNANCY
Safety for use in pregnancy has not been established.

Precautions
As with any potent drug, periodic assessment of renal, hepatic, and hematopoietic function should be made during prolonged therapy.

The possibility of superinfections with mycotic or bacterial pathogens should be kept in mind during therapy. If superinfections occur, appropriate therapy should be instituted.

Adverse Reactions
As with other penicillins, it may be expected that untoward reactions will be essentially limited to sensitivity phenomena. They are more likely to occur in individuals who have previously demonstrated hypersensitivity to penicillins and in those with a history of allergy, asthma, hay fever, or urticaria.

The following adverse reactions have been reported in association with ampicillin uses:

GASTROINTESTINAL: Glossitis, stomatitis, nausea, vomiting, diarrhea. (These reactions are usually associated with oral dosage forms.)

HYPERSENSITIVITY: Erythematous maculopapular rashes have been reported fairly frequently. Urticaria, erythema multiforme, and an occasional case of exfoliative dermatitis have been reported. Anaphylaxis is the most serious reaction experienced and has usually been associated with the parenteral dosage form.

NOTE: Urticaria, other skin rashes, and serum-sicknesslike reactions may be controlled with antihistamines and, if necessary, systemic corticosteroids. Whenever such reactions occur, ampicillin should be discontinued, unless, in the opinion of the physician, the condition being treated is life-threatening and amenable only to ampicillin therapy. Serious anaphylactoid reactions require the immediate use of epinephrine, oxygen, and intravenous steroids.

HEPATIC: A moderate rise in serum glutamic-oxaloacetic transaminase (SGOT) has been noted, particularly in infants, but the significance of this finding is unknown.

HEMIC AND LYMPHATIC: Anemia, thrombocytopenia, thrombocytopenic purpura, eosinophilia, leukopenia, and agranulocytosis have been reported during therapy with the penicillins. These reactions are usually reversible on discontinuation of therapy and are believed to be hypersensitivity phenomena.

Dosage (IM or IV)

Infection	Organisms	Adults	Children*
Respiratory tract	streptococci, pneumococci, nonpenicillinase-producing staphylococci, *H. influenzae*	250-500 mg q. 6 h.	25-50 mg/kg/day in equal doses q. 6 h.
Gastrointestinal tract	susceptible pathogens	500 mg q. 6 h.	50 mg/kg/day in equal doses q. 6 h.
Genitourinary tract	susceptible gram-negative or gram-positive pathogens	500 mg q. 6 h.	50 mg/kg/day in equal doses q. 6 h.
Urethritis (acute) in adult males	*N. gonorrhoeae*	500 mg b.i.d. for 1 day (IM)	
	(In complications such as prostatitis and epididymitis, prolonged and intensive therapy is recommended. Gonorrhea cases with suspected primary lesion of syphilis should have dark-field examinations before treatment. In any case suspected of concomitant syphilis, monthly serologic tests for at least 4 months are necessary.)		
Bacterial meningitis	*N. meningitidis, H. influenzae*	8-14 gram/day	100-200 mg/kg/day
	(Initial treatment is usually by IV drip, followed by frequent [q. 3-4 h.] IM injections.)		

*Children's dosage recommendations are intended for those whose weight will not result in a dosage higher than for the adult.

Smaller doses than those recommended in the table above should not be used. In stubborn or severe infections, therapy may be required for several weeks, and even higher doses may be needed. In treatment of chronic urinary or intestinal infections, frequent bacteriological and clinical appraisal is necessary, with follow-up for several months after cessation of therapy.

The treatment of gram-negative infections is often complicated by the emergence of resistant organisms (*Aerobacter aerogenes, Pseudomonas aeruginosa,* and others) which may cause superinfections. The possibility of such an occurrence should be kept in mind with use of ampicillin sodium.

Figure 8-12 *(Courtesy Wyeth Laboratories)*

Practice: Reading Labels

1. Figure 8-13—Circle the generic name and answer the following questions.
   a. What is the total amount of drug in the container? _____
   b. How many ml of diluting solution should be added to the vial for IM use? _____
   c. What is the dosage strength of the prepared solution? _____
2. Figure 8-14—Circle the trade name and answer the following questions.
   a. By what route(s) can this medication be given? _____
   b. How many ml of diluting solution should be added for IV administration? _____
   c. If 9.5 ml is added to the vial, how much of the resulting solution will contain 1 Gm? _____
3. Figure 8-15—Circle the total amount of drug in the vial and answer the following questions.
   a. By what route is this medication to be given? _____
   b. After reconstitution, where should the drug be stored? _____
   c. Assume the drug was reconstituted on 9/16. What would be the expiration date? _____
4. Figure 8-16—Circle the usual adult dosage and answer the following questions.
   a. How many ml of diluting solution should be added for IM use?
   _____
   b. How much of the resulting (reconstituted) solution is needed to administer 1 Gm of this medication? _____
   c. How long may the reconstituted solution be stored at room temperature? _____

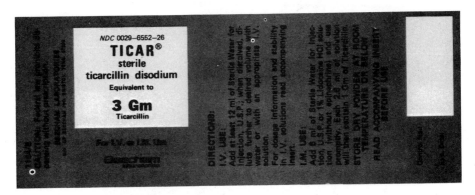

Figure 8-13 *(Courtesy Beecham Laboratories)*

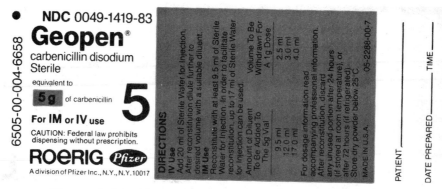

Figure 8-14   *(Courtesy Roerig, A Division of Pfizer Inc.)*

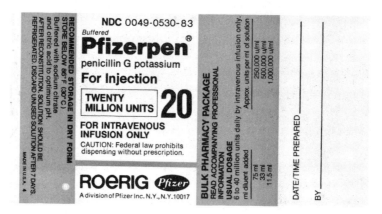

Figure 8-15   *(Courtesy Roerig, A Division of Pfizer Inc.)*

Figure 8-16   *(Courtesy Bristol-Myers U.S. Pharmaceutical Group, Evansville, IN 47721)*

5. Figure 8-17—Circle the route of administration and answer the following questions.
   a. How many mg of medication are contained in 2 ml? _____
   b. By what route only can this medication be given? _____
   c. What is the trade name of this drug? _____
6. Figure 8-18—Circle the usual adult dose and answer the following questions?
   a. How much solution should be added to administer this medication IV? _____
   b. What solution is used to prepare this medication for IV use?

   _____
   c. By which route(s) can this medication be given? _____
7. Figure 8-19—Circle the trade name and answer the following questions.
   The order is for Nembutal gr 1 ½.
   a. Is this a single or multiple dose container? _____
   b. How many grains are contained in this vial? _____
   c. How many mg are contained in this vial? _____
8. Figure 8-20—Circle the total amount contained in the vial and answer the following questions.
   a. What is the dosage strength of this medication? _____
   b. What is the generic name? _____
   c. Who manufactures this product? _____
9. Figure 8-21—Circle the generic name and answer the following questions.
   a. By what route *only* can the medication be given? _____
   b. Can the reconstituted solution be stored at room temperature?

   _____
   c. What is the total amount (volume) of solution in the vial?

   _____

(*Note:* See Appendix C for answer key.)

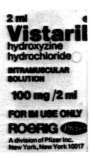

Figure 8-17 (*Courtesy Roerig, A Division of Pfizer Inc.*)

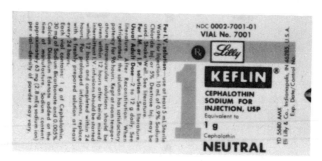

Figure 8-18   *(Courtesy Eli Lilly & Co.)*

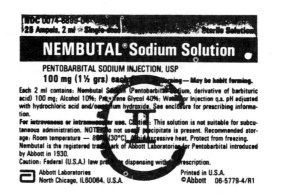

Figure 8-19   *(Courtesy Abbott Laboratories)*

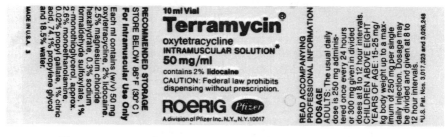

Figure 8-20   *(Courtesy Roerig, A Division of Pfizer Inc.)*

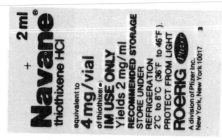

Figure 8-21   *(Courtesy Roerig, A Division of Pfizer Inc.)*

Calculating Dosages Obtained From Pre-Mixed Solutions

Many parenteral drugs are dispensed in vials or ampules that contain single or multiple doses. The label or printing on each container indicates the amount and the solution strength of the contents. Using these values as equivalents, the label factor method can be used to calculate the quantity of solution needed for the required dosage.

Examples:

a. A prescription order states: Atropine Sulfate gr $1/150$ IM. The vial of atropine (Figure 8-22) is labeled: Atropine Sulfate 0.4 mg per ml. How much solution will be administered?

Equivalents: gr 1 = 60 mg, 1 ml = 0.4 mg

$$\text{Conversion Equation:}\ \cancel{\text{gr}}\ 1/150 \times \frac{60\ \cancel{\text{mg}}}{\cancel{\text{gr}}\ 1} \times \frac{1\ \text{ml}}{0.4\ \cancel{\text{mg}}} = 1\ \text{ml}$$

OR

$$\cancel{\text{gr}}\ 0.007 \times \frac{60\ \cancel{\text{mg}}}{\cancel{\text{gr}}\ 1} \times \frac{1\ \text{ml}}{0.4\ \cancel{\text{mg}}} = 1.05 = 1.1\ \text{ml}$$

(*Note:* See pages 11–12 regarding answer discrepancies.)

b. The physician orders Demerol 20 mg IM. The medication is dispensed under the label Meperidine 50 mg/ml (Figure 8-23). Find the quantity of solution to be administered.

1. First: Consult a drug reference source to determine that Demerol is a brand name for the generic drug Meperidine.

2. Equivalents: 1 ml = 50 mg

$$\text{Conversion Equation:}\ 20\ \cancel{\text{mg}} \times \frac{1\ \text{ml}}{50\ \cancel{\text{mg}}} = 0.4\ \text{ml}$$

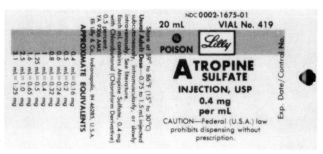

Figure 8-22 *(Courtesy Eli Lilly & Co.)*

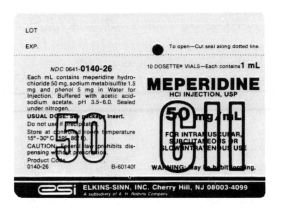

Figure 8-23 *(Courtesy Elkins-Sinn, Inc., A Subsidiary of A. H. Robins Company)*

c. Robinul 0.15 mg IM is ordered for the patient. On hand is a vial labeled: Robinul, (glycopyrrolate) 0.2 mg per ml (Figure 8-24). How many ml should be administered?
Equivalents: 0.2 mg = 1 ml

Conversion Equation: $0.15 \text{ mg} \times \dfrac{1 \text{ ml}}{0.2 \text{ mg}} = 0.8 \text{ ml}$

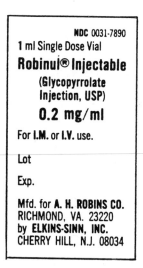

Figure 8-24 *(Courtesy Elkins-Sinn, Inc., A Subsidiary of A. H. Robins Company)*

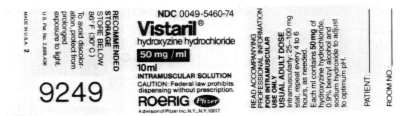

Figure 8-25 *(Courtesy Roerig, A Division of Pfizer Inc.)*

d. A patient is to receive Vistaril 35 mg IM. The medication comes in a vial labeled: Vistaril (hydroxyzine HCl) 50 mg per ml (Figure 8-25). Calculate the required dose to be administered in minims (use a tuberculin syringe).

Equivalents: 50 mg = 1 ml, 15 m = 1 ml

Conversion Equation: $35 \text{ mg} \times \dfrac{1 \text{ ml}}{50 \text{ mg}} \times \dfrac{15 \text{ m}}{1 \text{ ml}} = 10.5 \text{ m}$

Practice: Calculating Dosages from Pre-Mixed Solutions

(*Note:* Use the label factor method and calculate the correct dosage to be administered per dose. Carry each answer to two decimal places and round to nearest tenth.

1. **Order:** Meperidine 30 mg IM
   Label: Figure 8-26
   How many milliliters should be administered?

2. **Order:** Vistaril 75 mg IM
   Label: Figure 8-27. What is the generic name? _____
   How many milliliters should be administered?

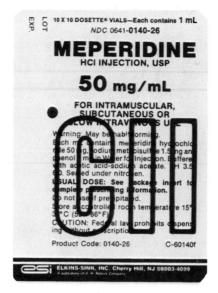

Figure 8-26 *(Courtesy Elkins-Sinn, Inc., A Subsidiary of A. H. Robins Company)*

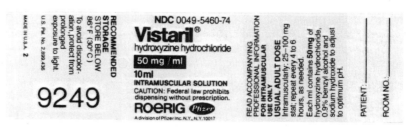

Figure 8-27 *(Courtesy Roerig, A Division of Pfizer Inc.)*

3. **Order:** Atropine Sulfate gr 1/100 IM
   Label: Figure 8-28
   How many milliliters should be administered?

4. **Order:** Robinul 0.1 mg IM
   Label: Figure 8-29. What is the generic name? _____
   How many milliliters should be administered?

5. **Order:** Duracillin 450,000 U IM
   Label: Figure 8-30. What is the generic name? _____
   How many milliliters should be administered?

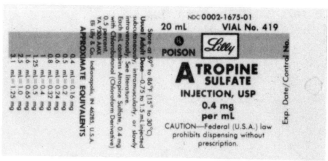

Figure 8-28   *(Courtesy Eli Lilly & Co.)*

NDC 0031-7890

1 ml Single Dose Vial

Robinul® Injectable

(Glycopyrrolate
Injection, USP)

0.2 mg/ml

For **I.M.** or **I.V.** use.

Lot

Exp.

Mfd. for **A. H. ROBINS CO.**
RICHMOND, VA. 23220
by **ELKINS-SINN, INC.**
CHERRY HILL, N.J. 08034

Figure 8-29 *(Courtesy Elkins-Sinn, Inc., A Subsidiary of A. H. Robins Company)*

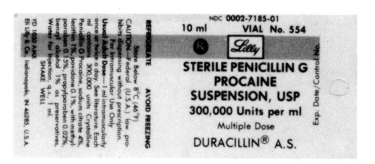

Figure 8-30 *(Courtesy Eli Lilly & Co.)*

6. **Order:** Omnipen-N 150 mg IM
   Label: Figure 8-31. What is the generic name? _____
   How many milliliters should be administered?

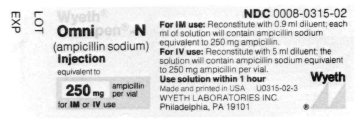

Figure 8-31   *(Courtesy Wyeth Laboratories)*

7. **Order:** Kantrex 150 mg IM
   Label: Figure 8-32 (3 ml = 1 Gm). What is the generic name?

   _____

   How many milliliters should be administered?

8. **Order:** Dramamine 35 mg IM
   Label: Figure 8-33. What is the generic name? _____
   How many milliliters should be administered?

9. **Order:** Digoxin 0.125 mg IM
   Label: Figure 8-34. What is the trade name? _____
   How many milliliters should be administered?

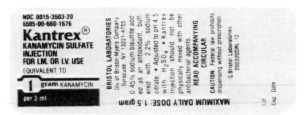

Figure 8-32   *(Courtesy Bristol-Myers U.S. Pharmaceutical Group, Evansville, IN 47721)*

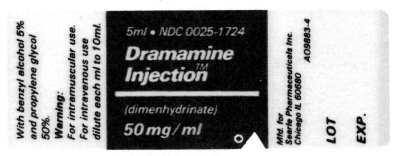

Figure 8-33   *(Courtesy G.D. Searle & Co.)*

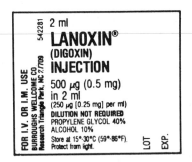

Figure 8-34   *(Courtesy Burroughs Wellcome Co.)*

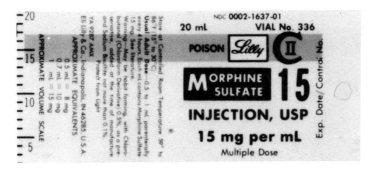

Figure 8-35 *(Courtesy Eli Lilly & Co.)*

10. **Order:** Morphine Sulfate gr ⅛
    Label: Figure 8-35
    How many milliliters should be administered?

Determine the number of milliliters that should be administered in the following problems. (Carry all answers to two decimal places and round to the nearest tenth.)

11. **Order:** Phenobarbitol Sodium 100 mg IM
    Label: Phenobarbital Sodium 125 mg/2 ml
    How many ml should be administered?

12. **Order:** Compazine 8 mg IM
    Label: Compazine (prochlorperazine) 10 mg/2 ml
    How many ml should be administered?

13. **Order:** Valium 4 mg IM
    Label: Valium (diazepam) 5 mg/ml

14. **Order:** Vitamin K 20 mg IM
    Label: Vitamin K 25 mg/2.5 cc

15. **Order:** Lanoxin 0.25 mg
    Label: Lanoxin (digoxin) 500 μg/2 ml

16. **Order:** Cedilanid-D 0.6 mg IM
    Label: Cedilanid-D (deslanoside) 0.8 mg/4 ml

17. **Order:** Phenergan 40 mg IM
    Label: Phenergan (promethazine) 50 mg/ml

18. **Order:** Adrenalin chloride 0.4 mg sc
    Label: Adrenalin chloride (epinephrine HCl) 1 mg/2 ml

19. **Order:** Garamycin 60 mg IM
    Label: Garamycin (gentamicin sulfate) 40 mg/ml

20. **Order:** Fentanyl Citrate Injection 0.05 mg IM
    Label: Fentanyl Citrate Injection 100 mcg/2 ml

(*Note:* See Appendix C for answer key.)

Calculations Based on Body Weight

The method for calculating oral dosages based on body weight was described in Unit 6. The method for calculating parenteral (IM or IV) dosages is identical.

Examples:

a. **Order:** Isoniazid Injection 5 mg/kg/day IM to an adult weighing 67 kg
   Label: Isoniazid Injection 100 mg/ml
   How many ml should be administered per dose?

$$67 \text{ kg} \times \frac{5 \text{ mg}}{1 \text{ kg}} \times \frac{1 \text{ ml}}{100 \text{ mg}} = 3.4 \text{ ml}$$

b. **Order:** Amikin 15 mg/kg/day IM in three divided doses to an adult weighing 155 lb
   Label: Amikin (amikacin) 500 mg/2 ml
   How many ml should be administered per dose?

$$155 \text{ lb} \times \frac{1 \text{ kg}}{2.2 \text{ lb}} \times \frac{15 \text{ mg}}{1 \text{ kg}} \times \frac{2 \text{ ml}}{500 \text{ mg}} = \frac{4.2 \text{ ml}}{3 \text{ doses}} = 1.4 \text{ ml/dose}$$

Practice: IM Calculations Based on Body Weight

1. **Order:** Gentamicin Sulfate 3 mg/kg/24 hr IM in three divided doses to an adult weighing 77 kg
   Label: Gentamicin Sulfate 40 mg/ml
   How many ml should be administered per dose?

2. **Order:** Neomycin Sulfate 15 mg/kg/dose IM to an adult weighing 120 lb
   Label: Neomycin Sulfate 250 mg/ml
   How many ml should be administered per dose?

3. **Order:** Kanamycin Sulfate Injection 15 mg/kg/24 hr IM in three divided doses to an adult weighing 60 kg
   Label: Kanamycin Sulfate Injection 0.5 Gm/2 ml
   How many ml should be administered per dose?

4. **Order:** Bretylol 5 mg/kg IM in four divided doses to an adult weighing 190 lb
   Label: Bretylol (bretylium tosylate) 1 Gm/20 ml
   How many ml should be administered per dose?

5. **Order:** Nebcin 3 mg/kg/dose IM to an adult weighing 80 kg
   Label: Nebcin (tobramycin sulfate) 80 mg/2 ml
   How many ml should be administered per dose?

6. **Order:** Benzquinamide 0.5 mg/kg/dose IM to an adult weighing 152 lb
   Label: Benzquinamide 25 mg/ml
   How many ml should be administered per dose?

7. **Order:** Amikacin Sulfate 15 mg/kg/day IM in two divided doses to an adult weighing 81.8 kg
   Label: Amikacin 500 mg/2 ml
   How many ml should be administered per dose?

8. **Order:** Kantrex Injection 15 mg/kg/day IM in four divided doses to an adult weighing 159 lb
   Label: Kantrex (kanamycin sulfate) Injection 1 Gm/3 ml
   How many ml should be administered per dose?

9. **Order:** Neobiotic 15 mg/kg IM in four divided doses to an adult weighing 78 kg
   Label: Neobiotic (neomycin sulfate) 250 mg/ml
   How many ml should be administered per dose?

10. **Order:** Nydrazid Injection 5 mg/kg/day IM in two divided doses to an adult weighing 128 lb
    Label: Nydrazid (isoniazid) Injection 100 mg/ml
    How many ml should be administered per dose?

(*Note:* See Appendix C for answer key.)

Units of Medication

Some drugs are measured in quantities called *units* (U). Unit quantities are frequently used for hormones, vitamins, antibiotics, antitoxins, and other biologicals. The value of a unit of drug is measured by the physiological effect a certain quantity will produce. Because the type of effect will vary for each drug, there is no common definition for a unit. Vials of these drugs may vary in strength from a few units to millions of units per ml. Because this information is on the label, the quantity of solution to be administered can be calculated using these given equivalents.

Because many of the drugs dispensed in units are extremely potent, dosages are often very small, requiring use of special syringes that can measure small doses. For example, the tuberculin syringe can measure quantities as small as 0.01 ml. Clinical calculations involving medications that will be measured in a tuberculin syringe should be carried to three decimal places and rounded to the nearest hundredth in the following manner:

- If the digit in the thousandths place is less than 5, this digit is dropped.
- If the digit in the thousandths place is 5 or greater, the hundredths digit is increased by one. For example:
  —0.256 ml; give 0.26 ml
  —0.382 ml; give 0.38 ml
  —0.615 ml; give 0.62 ml

The learner is reminded that insulin, which also is dispensed in units, should be measured only in an insulin syringe. Other medications that are ordered in larger quantities of units can be administered using a regular 2–3 cc syringe. The label factor method is used to convert units to milliliters or minims.

Example:

Order: H.P. Acthar Gel 50 U IM
Label: Figure 8-36
Dosage Strength: 80 U/ml

Conversion Equation: $50 \, \cancel{U} \times \dfrac{1 \, ml}{80 \, \cancel{U}} = 0.63 \, ml$

Practice: Medications Dispensed in Units

Determine the number of milliliters that should be administered in the following problems. (Carry all answers to two decimal places and round to the nearest tenth, unless the final digit is a 5.) Assume that dosages of less than 1 ml will be administered via tuberculin syringe.

1. **Order:** Vasopressin Injection 8 U IM
    Label: Figure 8-37

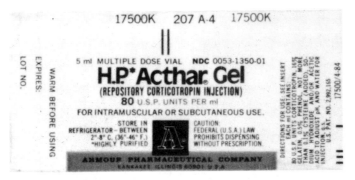

Figure 8-36 *(Courtesy Armour Pharmaceutical Company)*

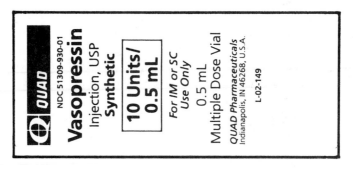

Figure 8-37   *(Courtesy QUAD Pharmaceuticals)*

2. **Order:** Heparin Sodium Injection 3500 U sc
   Label: Figure 8-38

3. **Order:** Tetanus Immune Globulin 200 U IM
   Label: Tetanus Immune Globulin 250 U/ml

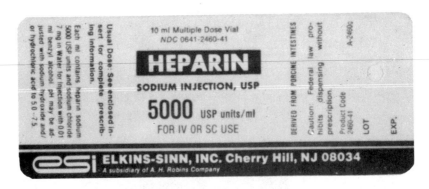

Figure 8-38 *(Courtesy Elkins-Sinn, Inc., A Subsidiary of A. H. Robins Company)*

4. **Order:** Wycillin 450,000 U IM
   Label: Wycillin (penicillin G procaine) 600,000 U/ml

5. **Order:** Penicillin G Benzathine 1,000,000 U IM
   Label: Penicillin G Benzathine 1,200,000 U/2 ml

6. **Order:** Tetanus Antitoxin 2500 U IM
   Label: Tetanus Antitoxin 1500 U/ml

7. **Order:** A.C.T.H. "80" Injectable 90 U IM
   Label: A.C.T.H. "80" (corticotropin) Injectable 400 U/5 ml

8. **Order:** BCG Vaccine 800,000 U ID
   Label: BCG Vaccine 8,000,000 U/ml

9. **Order:** Vitamin A 15,000 U IM
   Label: Vitamin A 50,000 U/ml

10. **Order:** Vitamin E 500 U IM
    Label: Vitamin E 200 U/ml

(*Note:* See Appendix C for answer key.)

Reconstitution of Drugs in Powder Form

Some medications are dispensed in vials containing the drug in dry powder form for reconstitution. These drugs lose their potency a short time after being placed in solution; therefore, they are not reconstituted until they are ready to be used.

A sterile diluent, usually either water or 0.9% sodium chloride (normal saline), must be added according to directions on the label or the manufacturer's package insert. This diluent must be labeled *Injection* or *For Injection,* Figure 8-39. Because other diluents may be specified on the label or accompanying circular (insert), be sure to read this information carefully. It is important that only diluents designated in the directions be used for reconstitution, because these have been determined to be compatible with the drug or the IV solution to which the drug will be added. For example, if the directions state, "Reconstitute only with sterile water for injection," do *not* substitute bacteriostatic water for injection; this contains preservatives that may alter the pH of the reconstituted solution and/or the effectiveness of the drug.

After the diluent is added, the vial must be shaken well to dissolve the powdered drug, which can then be drawn up into a syringe and

| STERILE WATER FOR INJECTION, USP | 0.9% SODIUM CHLORIDE INJECTION, USP |
| For Drug Diluent Use Only | For Drug Diluent Use Only |

Figure 8-39

administered. In some instances, the dissolved drug will expand the total resulting volume of solution. This must be taken into account when identifying equivalents; for example, the addition of 2 ml of diluent to a measured amount of dry drug may result in a total volume exceeding 2 ml. Therefore, it is necessary to refer to either the label or the package insert to ascertain the correct dosage strength or concentration of the reconstituted solution and to use the correct dosage strength in your calculation.

If the total amount of reconstituted medication is to be administered immediately (single dose vial), the expiration date need not be filled in, because the empty vial will be discarded. If the total amount of reconstituted medication is not to be administered immediately (multiple dose vial), the label or product insert will state how long the medication can be stored. This expiration date and/or time should then be written on the label, along with the initials of the person who reconstituted the drug.

Some reconstituted drugs can be frozen in individual doses and retain their potency for varying lengths of time. Once thawed, these drugs must be administered within a specified time period. Information regarding expiration date and/or time is found on the label or the package insert.

A Control (Lot) Number is stamped on the vial by the manufacturer. This refers to information regarding production and distribution of the drug.

Examples:

1. **Order:** Ticar (ticarcillin disodium) 500 mg IM
   Label: Figure 8-40; instructions for IM use
   - a. What diluent(s) should be used? *Sterile Water for Injection USP or 1% Lidocaine HCl Solution (without Epinephrine)*
   - b. How many ml should be added to the vial? __2 ml__
   - c. What is the dosage strength of the prepared solution? __2.6 ml = 1 Gm__
   - d. How many ml should the patient receive?

$$500 \ \text{mg} \times \frac{1 \ \text{Gm}}{1000 \ \text{mg}} \times \frac{2.6 \ \text{ml}}{1 \ \text{Gm}} = 1.3 \ \text{ml}$$

Some drug labels will indicate that various amounts of diluent can be added to the vial to yield various concentrations of solution, Figure 8-41. After the drug has been reconstituted, the strength of the resulting solution should be indicated on the label (check, underscore, circle, or write in the appropriate dilution). In addition, the expiration date should be noted and initialed so that the drug will not be used beyond its expiration date.

2. For each of the concentrations (dosage strength) listed on the label (Figure 8-41), how much diluent should be added to the vial and how

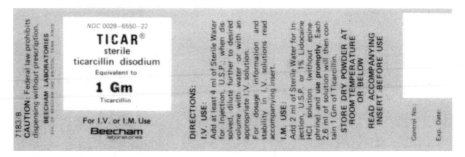

Figure 8-40 *(Courtesy Beecham Laboratories)*

much of the resulting solution would be administered to the patient if the order states: administer 600,000 U IM?

a. If 23 ml of diluent is added to the vial, the resulting solution will contain 200,000 U per ml.

   Dosage Strength: 1 ml = 200,000 U

   Conversion Equation: $600{,}000 \, \text{U} \times \dfrac{1 \, \text{ml}}{200{,}000 \, \text{U}} = 3 \, \text{ml}$

b. If 18 ml of diluent is added to the vial, the resulting solution will contain 250,000 U per ml.

   Dosage Strength: 1 ml = 250,000 U

   Conversion Equation: $600{,}000 \, \text{U} \times \dfrac{1 \, \text{ml}}{250{,}000 \, \text{U}} = 2.4 \, \text{ml}$

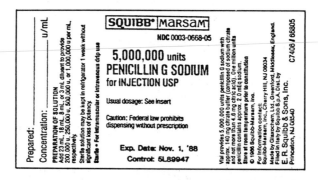

Figure 8-41 *(Courtesy E. R. Squibb & Sons, Inc.)*

c. If 8 ml of diluent is added to the vial, the resulting solution will contain 500,000 U per ml.
Dosage Strength: 1 ml = 500,000 U

Conversion Equation: $600,000 \text{ U} \times \dfrac{1 \text{ ml}}{500,000 \text{ U}} = 1.2 \text{ ml}$

d. If 3 ml of diluent is added to the vial, the resulting solution will contain 1,000,000 U per ml.
Dosage Strength: 1 ml = 1,000,000 U

Conversion Equation: $600,000 \text{ U} \times \dfrac{1 \text{ ml}}{1,000,000 \text{ U}} = 0.6 \text{ ml}$

e. How long may the reconstituted solution be stored? __7 days__
f. Where should it be stored? __refrigerator__

Practice: Reconstitution of Drugs in Powder Form

1. **Order:** Polycillin-N 350 mg IM
   Label: Figure 8-42; instructions for IM use. What is the generic name? _____
   a. How many ml should be added to the vial? _____
   b. How will you know what diluent to add? _____
   c. What is the dosage strength of the resulting solution? _____
   d. How soon must this solution be administered? _____
   e. How many ml should the patient receive? _____
   f. What is the usual adult dosage of this drug? _____
2. **Order:** Prostaphlin 300 mg IM
   Label: Figure 8-43; instructions for IM use. What is the generic name? _____
   a. What diluent should be used for reconstitution? _____
   b. How much diluent should be added to the vial? _____
   c. What is the dosage strength of the prepared solution? _____
   d. How many ml should the patient receive? _____
   e. What is the usual adult dose of this drug? _____
   f. Assume you reconstituted the drug at 10 A.M. on 9/16. What is the expiration time/date:
      ■ if you stored the vial at room temperature? _____
      ■ if you refrigerated the vial? _____
3. **Order:** Geopen 500 mg IM
   Label: Figure 8-44; instructions for IM use. What is the generic name? _____
   a. What diluent should be added to the vial? _____
   b. Assume you added 4 ml of diluent; what is the resulting dosage strength?

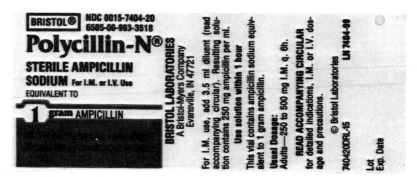

Figure 8-42 *(Courtesy Bristol-Myers U.S. Pharmaceutical Group, Evansville, IN 47721)*

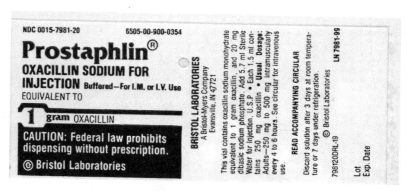

Figure 8-43 *(Courtesy Bristol-Myers U.S. Pharmaceutical Group, Evansville, IN 47721)*

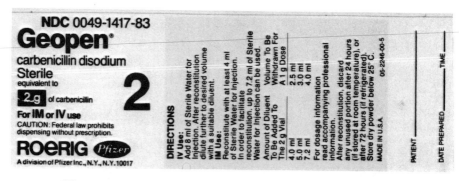

Figure 8-44 *(Courtesy Roerig, A Division of Pfizer Inc.)*

   c. How soon must this reconstituted medication be administered:
- ■ at room temperature? _____
- ■ if refrigerated? _____

   d. How many ml should the patient receive? _____

   e. How can you compare the usual adult dosage with the dosage ordered for this patient? _____

4. **Order:** Keflin 500 mg IM q 6 h

   Label: Figure 8-45; instructions for IM use: Each Gm should be diluted with 4 ml Sterile Water for Injection to yield a concentration of 0.5 Gm/2.2 ml. What is the generic name?

   _____

   a. What diluent should be added to the vial? _____

   b. How much diluent should be added to the vial? _____

   c. What is the dosage strength of the prepared solution? _____

   d. How many ml should the patient receive per dose? _____

   e. How many Gm would this patient receive over a 24 hr period?

   _____

   f. What is the usual adult dose of this drug? _____

   g. Assume you reconstituted the drug at 9 A.M. on 11/9. What is the expiration time/date if the solution is stored in the refrigerator?

   _____

   h. How soon after reconstitution must the medication be administered if it is not refrigerated? _____

5. **Order:** Penicillin G Potassium 400,000 U IM qid

   For each concentration (dosage strength) listed on the label (Figure 8-46), calculate the number of ml the patient should receive.

   a. If 9.6 ml of diluent is added to the vial:

   Dosage Strength:

   Conversion Equation:

   b. If 4.6 ml of diluent is added to the vial:

   Dosage Strength:

   Conversion Equation:

   c. If 3.6 ml of diluent is added to the vial:

   Dosage Strength:

   Conversion Equation:

   d. How long may the reconstituted solution be stored? _____

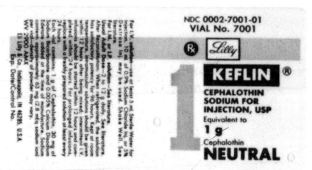

Figure 8-45   *(Courtesy Eli Lilly & Co.)*

   e. Where should the solution be stored? _____

   f. What is the usual IM dosage of this drug? _____

   g. How does the above ordered dosage compare with the usual IM dosage of this drug? _____

    Determine the number of milliliters that should be administered in the following problems. (Carry all answers to two decimal places and round to the nearest tenth.)

6. **Order:** Ampicillin 150 mg IM
   Label: Ampicillin 500 mg—multiple dose vial
   Reconstitution: Add 1.8 ml of sterile diluent to yield 250 mg/ml

Figure 8-46   *(Courtesy E. R. Squibb & Sons, Inc.)*

7. **Order:** Pipracil 800 mg IM
   Label: Pipracil (piperacillin sodium) 1 Gm powder form
   Reconstitution: Add 2 ml of sterile diluent to yield 1 Gm/2.5 ml

8. **Order:** Keflin 500 mg IM
   Label: Keflin (cephalothin) 1 Gm
   Reconstitution: Add 4 ml of sterile diluent to yield 0.5 Gm/2.2 ml

9. **Order:** Penicillin G Potassium 500,000 U IM
   Label: Penicillin G Potassium 1,000,000 U/vial
   Reconstitution: Add 4.6 ml of sterile diluent to yield 200,000 U/ml

10. **Order:** Geopen 1 Gm IM
    Label: Geopen (carbexicillin disodium) 5 Gm
    Reconstitution: Add 7 ml of sterile diluent to yield 1 Gm/2 ml

11. **Order:** Polycillin-N 250 mg IM
    Label: Polycillin-N (ampicillin sodium) 1 Gm in dry form
    Reconstitution: Add 3.5 ml of sterile diluent to yield 250 mg/ml

12. **Order:** Unipen 400 mg IM
    Label: Unipen (nafcillin sodium) 1 Gm in powder form
    Reconstitution: Add 3.4 ml sterile water for injection to yield 4 ml/Gm

13. **Order:** Ampicillin 500 mg IM
    Label: Ampicillin 1 Gm/vial in dry form
    Reconstitution: Add 1.8 ml sterile water to yield to 250 mg/ml

14. **Order:** Staphcillin 1.5 Gm IM
    Label: Staphcillin (methicillin sodium) 6 Gm vial in dry form
    Reconstitution: Add 8.6 ml of sterile normal saline to yield 500 mg/ml

15. **Order:** Streptomycin 1 Gm IM
    Label: Streptomycin 5 Gm in dry form
    Reconstitution: Add 9.0 ml of sterile water to yield 400 mg/ml

16. **Order:** Keflin 1 Gm IM
    Label: Keflin (cephalothin) 1 Gm in dry form
    Reconstitution: Add 4 ml of sterile water to yield 0.5 Gm/2.2 ml

17. **Order:** Penicillin G Sodium 300,000 U IM
    Label: Penicillin G Sodium 1,000,000 U/vial in dry form
    Reconstitution: Add 4.6 ml of sterile diluent to provide 200,000 U/ml

18. **Order:** Prostaphlin 150 mg IM
    Label: Prostaphlin (oxacillin sodium) 0.5 Gm/vial in dry form
    Reconstitution: Add 2.7 ml of sterile water to yield 250 mg/1.5 ml

19. **Order:** Ampicillin 350 mg IM
    Label: Ampicillin 0.5 Gm/vial in dry form
    Reconstitution: Add 2.7 ml of sterile water to yield a concentration
    of 250 mg/1.5 ml

20. **Order:** Penicillin G Benzathine 400,000 U IM
    Label: Penicillin G Benzathine 1,000,000 U/vial in dry form
    Reconstitution: Add 3.6 ml sterile diluent to yield 250,000 U/ml

(*Note:* See Appendix C for answer key.)

Administration of Parenteral Medications

···

Objectives

Upon completion of this unit of study you should be able to:
- *Identify safe and suitable sites for intradermal, subcutaneous, and intramuscular injections, including boundaries and anatomical landmarks.*
- *Follow infection-control guidelines with respect to handling or manipulating needles and syringes.*
- *List the general rules for safe administration of parenteral medications: preparing, administering, and recording.*
- *Identify performance criteria related to administering drugs by subcutaneous and intramuscular routes, including variations when administering heparin and insulin.*
- *Read drug labels to differentiate various types of insulin.*

Injection Sites and Techniques

A descriptive overview of injection sites and procedures follows, along with recommended guidelines for administration of parenteral medications. For detailed instruction on injection techniques, the learner is referred to a pharmacology or nursing text.

Intradermal Injection

Intradermal administration is the introduction of medication into the dermal layers of the skin. The needle penetrates the epidermis and enters the dermis. A very small amount of drug is given, usually for the purpose of skin testing. A 1 cc tuberculin syringe is used with a fine (25–26) gauge, 1/4″–5/8″ needle. The medial surface of the forearm and the upper chest and back are the most commonly used sites, Figure 9-1. A very shallow angle of insertion, 10–15°, is used. The needle is inserted bevel up through the tautly held skin so that it is visible just beneath the surface and the

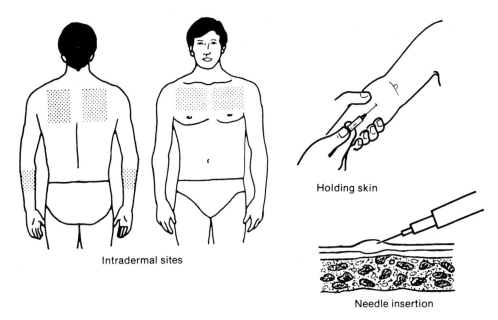

Intradermal sites

Holding skin

Needle insertion

Figure 9-1 Intradermal injections

medication is injected slowly until a small wheal is produced. Aspiration prior to injection is omitted. The needle is removed and the site wiped gently so as not to disperse the medication; the area is not massaged for the same reason. A bandage should not be applied and the patient should be instructed not to scratch or rub the site.

Subcutaneous Injection

Subcutaneous injection is the introduction of medication into the subcutaneous layer of connective and fatty tissue. Because this layer lies directly beneath the dermis, small amounts of solution are injected, usually not more than 2 ml in a site. A 1–3 ml syringe is used with a 25–28 gauge, 1/2″–5/8″ needle. Shorter or longer needles may be employed depending on the size and/or obesity of the recipient. When a 1/2″ needle is used, the needle is inserted at a 90° angle; with a 5/8″–1″ needle, the angle of insertion is 45°, Figure 9-2. Subcutaneous injections may be administered at any site where there is an adequate layer of subcutaneous tissue. The most commonly used sites are: the upper outer arms, the anterior or lateral thighs, the abdomen from below the costal margins to the iliac crest (one and a half to two inches away from the umbilicus), the upper back below the scapulae, and the subcutaneous tissue over the dorsogluteal area. The areas over the deltoid and vastus lateralis or rectus femoris muscles often are used as long as the subcutaneous tissue can

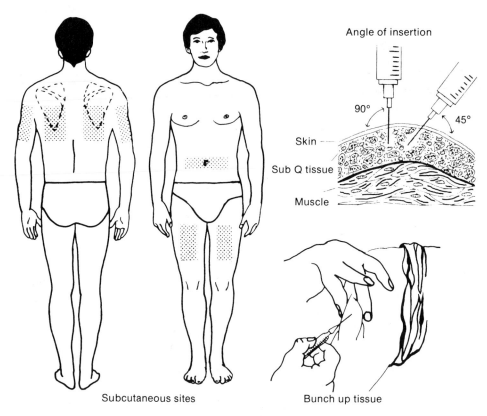

Angle of insertion

90°

45°

Skin

Sub Q tissue

Muscle

Subcutaneous sites   Bunch up tissue

Figure 9-2   Subcutaneous injections

be bunched up so that the needle does not enter the muscle. When frequent subcutaneous injections are administered—such as daily insulin injections—a plan should be devised for rotating sites to promote absorption and avoid tissue fibrosis. Aspiration usually is performed prior to injection to avoid the possibility of intravascular injection, but there are exceptions to this rule. For example: persons with diabetes who self-administer insulin are no longer being taught to aspirate, for the purpose of facilitating this procedure. An inadvertent intravenous administration of insulin is not considered harmful. In the case of heparin, aspiration also is omitted, because of the possibility of tissue damage with resulting subcutaneous bleeding. The nurse always should ascertain whether aspiration is required or contraindicated when administering subcutaneous injections.

Intramuscular Injection

Intramuscular administration of medications is made through the skin and subcutaneous tissues into a muscle, Figure 9-3. Sites must be chosen

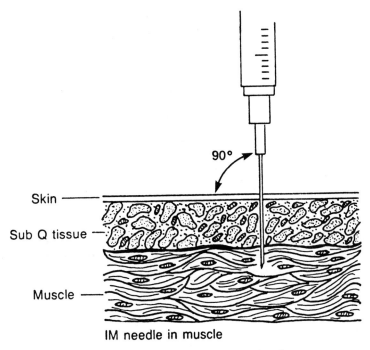

Skin

Sub Q tissue

Muscle

90°

IM needle in muscle

Figure 9-3 Intramuscular injections

with care to avoid damage to major nerves and blood vessels either by the needle or the medication. The most commonly used sites are the gluteal muscles. Also used are the deltoid, the vastus lateralis, and the rectus femoris. The sites should be rotated when the medication is irritating or repeated frequently.

The size of syringe and needle chosen depends on the amount and viscosity of medication to be given and the size and/or obesity of the recipient. For aqueous solutions, a 21 or 22 gauge, 1″–1 ½″ needle is usually suitable. For viscous or oily solutions, a 20 or 21 gauge needle of appropriate length is used. For both a 90° angle of insertion is used.

It is necessary to aspirate prior to injection of the medication to avoid inadvertent intravenous injection. Following injection of most medications, the area is massaged gently to aid dispersion and absorption. The nurse always should ascertain the correct procedure regarding massage when intramuscular medications are administered.

Ventrogluteal Site This site utilizes the ventral area of the gluteal muscles, specifically, the gluteus medius and minimus muscles below the iliac crest. These muscles can absorb up to 3 ml of solution per injection.

This versatile site can be used with the patient in a lateral, supine, or prone position or—less desirable but possible—with the person standing or seated. Three anatomical landmarks are used to identify the site. The palm of the hand is placed on the greater trochanter of the femur, the index finger on the anterior superior iliac spine, and the middle finger abducted posteriorly along the iliac crest to form a V-shaped area. The injection site is in the center of the triangle between the index and middle fingers, Figure 9-4.

This is a safe injection site for both adults and for children over the age of 1 year. It is particularly useful in the case of small or emaciated persons, because the muscle layer is thick and easily accessible.

Dorsogluteal Site   The dorsogluteal site is located in the upper, outer quadrant of the buttock. Injection is made into the gluteus maximus muscle, which also can absorb up to 3 ml of solution. There are two methods for locating the dorsogluteal site using anatomical landmarks. The patient may be positioned on one side or the other or on the abdomen with the toes pointed inward. For method one: the buttock is divided into imaginary quadrants using a vertical line extending from the crest of the ilium to the gluteal fold and a horizontal line from the top of the medial fold to the lateral border. The injection site is in the upper, outer quadrant about 2–3 inches below the iliac crest. For method two: the posterior iliac spine is palpated, as is the greater trochanter of the femur, and an imaginary line is drawn between these two points. The injection site is

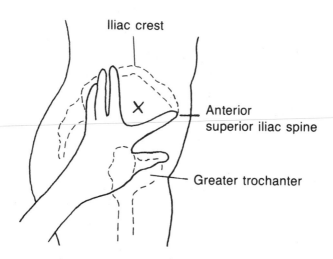

Figure 9-4   Ventrogluteal site

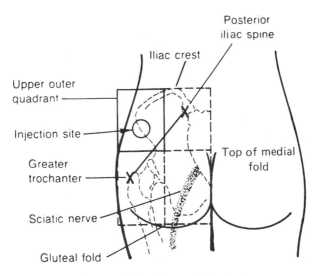

Figure 9-5 Dorsogluteal site

lateral and superior to this line, Figure 9-5. The gluteal muscle is not used for infants, because it is small and poorly developed. The site may be used by the age of 3 years for children who have been walking at least a year.

Deltoid Site   The recommended site of injection into the deltoid muscle is into the thicker mid-portion of the muscle. This is a relatively small area and is used when small amounts of solution are to be given, not exceeding 2 ml in adults. Because the deltoid muscle is very thin in infants and children, it is used only when very small amounts, not exceeding 0.5 ml, are to be given. The patient may be positioned on either side or sitting up. It is important that the arm hang loosely at the side when the patient is seated because this keeps the muscle relaxed. Holding the arm away from the body tenses the muscle and increases discomfort as well as impeding dispersion of the medication. The anatomical landmarks for identification of the deltoid site include the acromion process of the scapula and the axillary fold. The site is located at the center of the triangular area bounded superiorly by the acromion process and inferiorly by a line extending from the axillary fold across the lateral aspect of the arm, Figure 9-6.

Vastus Lateralis Site   The vastus lateralis muscle is a commonly used injection site, because it is usually thick and well developed in both adults

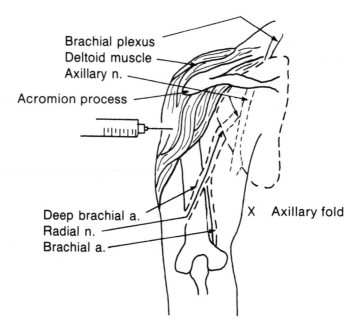

Figure 9-6 Deltoid site

and children. The site can absorb up to 3 ml of solution, depending on the size of the individual. The patient may be in a lateral or supine position or sitting upright. The anatomical landmarks for identification of the site are the knee and the greater trochanter of the femur. Injection is made into the mid-portion of the muscle, located by measuring a hand's width above the knee and below the trochanter. The muscle extends from the mid-anterior to mid-lateral thigh between the two bony landmarks, Figure 9-7.

Rectus Femoris Site   The rectus femoris muscle, on the anterior aspect of the thigh, can be used for intramuscular injections of up to 3 ml and is especially accessible for individuals who self-administer their injections. The patient assumes a sitting or lying position and the injection site is in the lateral mid-portion of the anterior thigh. The medial aspect of the thigh should be avoided, Figure 9-8.

Precautions in Handling Needles and Syringes

Because of the risk associated with contacting blood contaminated with microorganisms, personnel must use special precautions when handling all used needles and syringes. It is recommended that a glove be placed

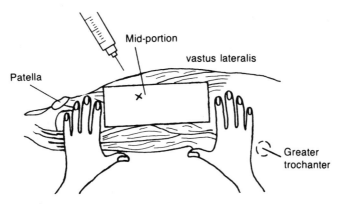

Figure 9-7 Vastus lateralis site

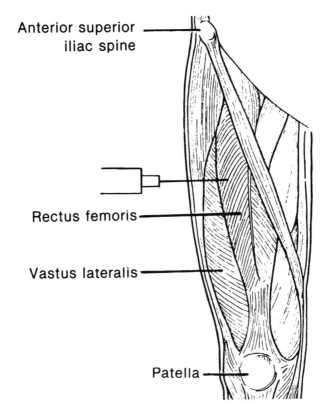

Figure 9-8 Rectus femoris site

on the non-dominant hand (i.e., the hand that comes into contact with the patient) when any injection is administered. In addition, because of the danger of needle-stick injuries, used needles should not be recapped, bent, or broken following injection. They should not be removed from disposable syringes or otherwise manipulated by hand. All used needles and syringes should immediately be discarded into puncture-resistant containers. Personnel should ascertain agency policy with regard to handling and disposing of syringes and needles, and they should follow these guidelines meticulously. Any time gloves are worn when handling needles and syringes, hands should be washed thoroughly immediately after gloves are removed, even if the gloves appear to be intact.

Administration of Parenteral Medications

The general rules for administration of medications, which were listed in Unit 7, also apply here. Because of the additional potential for harm to the patient when medications are given parenterally, accuracy and care in preparing and administering these drugs assumes critical proportions. Precise identification of sites and proper techniques of administration cannot be overemphasized. Principles of safety, comfort, and effective intervention are equally important.

In addition to the rules in Unit 7, specific recommendations for administration of intradermal, subcutaneous, and intramuscular injections include:

- Select a sterile syringe and needle of the appropriate size and length.
- Mix solution in vial, if necessary, by rotating between palms or shaking gently.
- If irritating medications are being administered, it is desirable to change the needle after obtaining the correct dose.
- Carefully select and identify injection sites by fully exposing area and palpating anatomical landmarks.
- Rotate injection sites as appropriate for repeated injections. A chart or diagram for rotation of injection sites is often desirable.
- Obtain assistance as necessary if patient needs to be restrained.
- Place glove on non-dominant hand.
- Cleanse skin at the injection site with an antiseptic wipe.
- Hold syringe in one hand; with the other hand bunch or hold the skin taut at the injection site, as appropriate for type of injection and angle of insertion.
- Insert the needle about seven eighths of its length, thus preventing complete disappearance in case of breakage.
- Aspirate for blood to avoid an accidental intravascular injection. If blood is aspirated, remove the needle, obtain a new needle, syringe, and dose and select a new site. Aspiration is omitted with intradermal

injections and certain subcutaneous medications (i.e., insulin, heparin).

■ Inject the medication into the tissue with slow, steady pressure.

■ For IM injection, place the antiseptic wipe adjacent to the needle, apply reverse pressure, and quickly withdraw the needle, immediately making slight pressure over the site with the wipe.

■ For subcutaneous injection: (longer needle, 45° angle), lay the antiseptic wipe over the injection site without exerting pressure on the needle, quickly remove the needle, and then apply pressure over the site; (shorter needle, 90° angle), proceed as in IM injection above.

■ Gently massage the injection site with an antiseptic wipe to increase the rate of dispersion and absorption. Avoid massage with intradermal, insulin, heparin, or Z-track.

■ Discard used syringe and needle (without re-capping) into puncture-resistant container.

The learner may find the following checklist a helpful guide for the administration of parenteral medications.

Performance Criteria: Administration of Injections

	S	U	Comments
A. Preparing the medication 1. Obtains medication Medex to confirm medication order regarding dose, route, and time of administration			
2. Checks for any known allergies			
3. Washes hands			
4. Selects appropriate size syringe and needle a) Intradermal injection: 1 cc tuberculin syringe with 25–27 gauge, 1/4″ to 5/8″ needle			
b) Subcutaneous injection: 1–3 cc syringe with 25–28 gauge, 1/2″ to 1″ needle			
c) Intramuscular injection: 1–3 cc syringe with 20–22 gauge, 1″ to 1 1/2″ needle			

Continued on next page

Performance Criteria: Administration of Injections (Cont.)

	S	U	Comments
5. Obtains correct medication (vial, ampule, or cartridge)			
6. Checks medication label against Medex			
7. Checks for expiration date of medication			
8. Withdraws medication into syringe a) *Vial:* 1. cleanses stopper with antiseptic wipe			
2. injects air into vial equal to amount of medication to be withdrawn			
3. withdraws accurate dosage of medication, changes needle where appropriate			
b) *Glass Ampule:* 1. wraps ampule in gauze or antiseptic wipe			
2. snaps off top of ampule			
3. places needle into open ampule and withdraws required dosage			
c) *Double Vial Technique:* (Mixing two medications in one syringe) 1. cleanses stoppers on both vials with antiseptic wipe			
2. placing first vial on a flat surface, injects air into air space equal to the desired dose			
3. injects air into second vial equal to the desired dose and then withdraws this amount of medication			
4. recleanses top of first vial, reinserts needle, and withdraws de-			

Continued on next page

Performance Criteria: Administration of Injections (Cont.)

	S	U	Comments
sired dose, being careful not to inject any medication from second vial			
5. returns or disposes of drug container properly			
6. re-checks labels against the Medex			
d) *Pre-Filled cartridge:* 1. Inserts into cartridge holder			
2. Ejects excess air			

B. Administering the injection
   1. *Intradermal*
   a) Identifies the correct patient			

b) Selects correct site —ventral forearm			
—upper chest area			
—sub-scapular area			
c) Places glove on non-dominant hand			
d) Cleanses site with antiseptic wipe and allows to dry			
e) Spreads the site to hold tissue taut			
f) Positions syringe so needle is at 10° to 15° angle to the patient's skin; bevel up			
g) Inserts needle ⅛″ below skin's surface with point visible through skin			
h) Injects medication slowly until wheal forms			

Continued on next page

Performance Criteria: Administration of Injections (Cont.)

	S	U	Comments
i) Withdraws needle, blots gently with antiseptic wipe, avoiding massage			
j) Places used syringe and needle (without re-capping) into puncture-resistant container			
2. *Subcutaneous* a) Identifies correct patient			
b) Provides privacy			
c) Selects correct site —outer aspects of upper arms			
—anterior and outer aspects of thighs			
—abdomen, above iliac crests (1 ½–2″ away from umbilicus)			
—sub-scapular region of back —dorso-ventrogluteal area			
d) Places glove on non-dominant hand			
e) Cleanses site with antiseptic wipe			
f) Grasps skin between thumb and forefinger to elevate subcutaneous tissue			
g) Inserts ½″ needle at 90° angle to skin and ⅝″ or longer needle at 45° angle with bevel up			
h) Releases skin and grasps hub of syringe to stabilize needle			
i) Aspirates for blood, keeping needle and syringe steady. If blood appears, withdraws needle, discards medication, obtains new syringe, needle, and dose, and selects new site			

Continued on next page

Performance Criteria: Administration of Injections (Cont.)

	S	U	Comments
j) Injects medication slowly			
k) Places antiseptic wipe over (45°) or adjacent to (90°) the needle without applying pressure			
l) Removes needle quickly and immediately applies pressure with antiseptic wipe			
m) Massages site gently, unless contraindicated			
n) Discards used syringe and needle (without re-capping) into puncture-resistance container			
3. *Intramuscular* a) Identifies correct patient			
b) Provides privacy			
c) Selects correct site —ventrogluteal			
—dorsogluteal			
—deltoid			
—vastus lateralis			
—rectus femoris			
d) Places glove on non-dominant hand			
e) Positions patient and exposes site			
f) Cleanses site with antiseptic wipe			
g) Stretches skin taut at injection site			
h) Quickly injects needle at 90° angle, using a dart-like thrust			

Continued on next page

Performance Criteria: Administration of Injections (Cont.)

	S	U	Comments
i) Releases stretched skin and grasps hub of syringe to stabilize needle			
j) Aspirates for blood, keeping needle and syringe steady. If blood appears, withdraws needle, discards medication, obtains new syringe, needle, and dose, and selects a new site			
k) Injects medication slowly			
l) Places antiseptic wipe adjacent to site			
m) Withdraws needle quickly and immediately applies antiseptic wipe			
n) Massages site gently, unless contraindicated			
o) Discards used syringe and needle (without re-capping) into puncture-resistant container			
C. Following injection 1. Leaves patient comfortable			
2. Disposes of equipment according to hospital policy			
3. Records accurately			
D. Maintains principles of asepsis throughout the procedure			
E. Maintains principles of patient safety and comfort throughout the procedure			

S—Satisfactory   U—Unsatisfactory   Evaluator _____

Variation of Parenteral Injection Techniques: IM

Z-Track

This is a method of administering a deep intramuscular injection to prevent seepage of medication along the needle track. The method is used when any medication that is irritating or a substance that stains such as iron is given, because it is more effective in sealing medication within the desired site than the customary (usual) intramuscular injection technique. Figure 9-9 illustrates the technique of Z-track injection.

It is important to select a deep site in a large muscle, preferably the dorsogluteal site. See Figure 9-9. It is also important to apply a new needle after obtaining the desired dose to prevent depositing medication in the subcutaneous tissues as the needle is inserted into the muscle. In addition, a 0.5 ml air lock is used to clear the needle of medication after injection and to help prevent leakage or tracking. Therefore, after the correct dosage is obtained, 0.5 ml of air is drawn into the syringe to provide the desired air lock following injection of the medication.

Performance Criteria: Z-Track Method—Deep Intramuscular Injection

(*Note:* Follows usual procedure for intramuscular injection with the following modifications.)

	S	U	Comments
1. Selects appropriate size syringe with suitable needle for withdrawing medication. (This needle will be discarded.)			
2. After obtaining medication, pulls back plunger to add 0.5 ml air lock			
3. Replaces needle with sterile needle, 20 or 21 gauge, 1 ¼"–1 ½" long (for iron—19 or 20 gauge, 2"–3" long)			
4. Uses dorsogluteal site (this is the only acceptable site)			
5. Places glove on non-dominant hand			
6. Displaces skin firmly to one side, then cleanses selected site with antiseptic wipe			
7. Inserts needle at 90° angle			

Continued on next page

Performance Criteria: Z-Track Method—Deep Intramuscular Injection (Cont.

	S	U	Comments
8. While maintaining retracted skin, aspirates for blood, then injects medication slowly			
9. Waits 10 seconds (still maintaining skin retraction)			
10. Withdraws needle quickly, simultaneously releasing retracted skin			
11. Does *NOT* massage site			
12. Discards used syringe and needle (without re-capping) into puncture-resistant container			
13. Records location of injection site (rotates site)			

S—Satisfactory   U—Unsatisfactory   Evaluator _____

In the Z-track technique, the skin and subcutaneous tissues are displaced to one side, resulting in a shift of tissue layers out of normal alignment (see Figure 9-9). The needle is inserted directly into the muscle layer and the medication is injected slowly while tissue displacement is maintained. It is therefore necessary to aspirate and hold the syringe

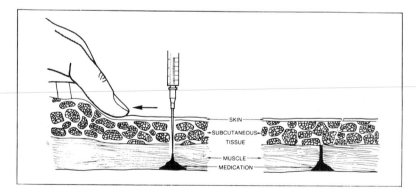

Figure 9-9 The Z-track technique for deep intramuscular injection *(Courtesy of Reiss and Melick,* Pharmacological Aspects of Nursing Care, Second Edition. *Copyright 1987 by Delmar Publishers Inc.)*

with the same hand. A period of 10 seconds is allowed to elapse before needle removal to assure adequate dispersion. When the needle is removed, the tissues are quickly released and return to their normal position, leaving a Z-shaped channel that prevents seepage and tracking. The site is not massaged.

The checklist on pp. 147–148 may be used as a guide for the Z-track variation.

Variation of Parenteral Injection Techniques: SC

Heparin Injection

Subcutaneous injection of heparin requires special modifications in technique to cause as little trauma as possible to the tissues at the injection site. The purpose is to prevent or minimize bleeding caused by the anticoagulant properties of this drug. To avoid inadvertent intramuscular injection, it is important to select a short needle and a site with adequate subcutaneous tissue. Separate needles should be used for obtaining and injecting the heparin. Sites on the abdomen above the level of the anterior iliac spines are most commonly used, Figure 9-10. It is important to rotate sites and to select sites free from bruising or scarring and at least 2″ away from the umbilicus. Gentle cleansing of the skin helps prevent trauma, as does omission of aspiration and massage. The patient also should be reminded not to rub the site. Application of an icebag following injection may prevent ecchymosis.

The following checklist may be used as a guide for the heparin injection.

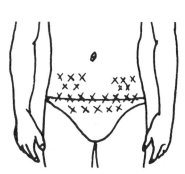

Figure 9-10   Heparin sites

Performance Criteria: Administration of Heparin

(*Note:* Follows usual procedure for subcutaneous injection with the following modifications.)

	S	U	Comments
1. Selects appropriate size syringe with 25–27 gauge needle, $\frac{1}{2}''$–$\frac{5}{8}''$ long plus second sterile needle for injection			
2. Obtains correct dose and changes needle			
3. Selects correct site: abdomen, above the anterior iliac spines and 2″ away from umbilicus, scars, or ecchymoses			
4. Places glove on non-dominant hand			
5. Gently bunches a well-defined roll of tissue without pinching			
6. Wipes site with antiseptic wipe (avoids rubbing)			
7. While maintaining roll, inserts needle at a 90° angle into subcutaneous fatty tissue. Does *NOT* aspirate for blood. While still maintaining roll of tissue and keeping needle steady, slowly injects medication			
8. Withdraws needle in same direction of insertion while simultaneously releasing tissue roll			
9. Holds antiseptic wipe at injection site for $\frac{1}{2}$–1 minute. Does *NOT* massage site			
10. Discards used syringe and needle (without re-capping) into puncture-resistant container			
11. Records location of injection site (rotates injection sites)			

S—Satisfactory   U—Unsatisfactory   Evaluator _____

Insulin Preparations

Persons who have diabetes caused by insulin-secretion deficiency may be treated by regular (daily or more often) injections of manufactured insulin. Sources of manufactured insulin are: pork pancreas, beef pancreas, or a combination of the two. Synthetic human insulin is also available. Because allergic reactions are possible, alternative forms of insulin may be prescribed. If the source is identified in the insulin order, it is essential that the correct bottle be selected, Figure 9-11.

Insulins differ as to time of onset, peak of activity, and duration of action. These characteristics are controlled by adding zinc and/or protamine to regular (fast-acting) insulin to produce either intermediate or long-acting effects. These extended-action products are called *modified* insulin and are designated by the letters S, L, N, P, and U.

Regular insulin is a clear solution designated by the letter R on the bottle. An example is shown in Figure 9-11. It can be administered subcu-

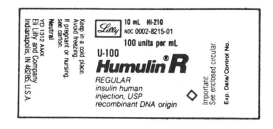

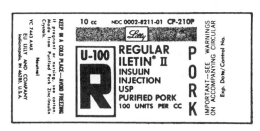

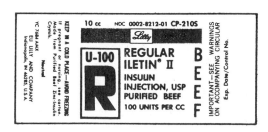

Figure 9-11 *(Courtesy Eli Lilly & Co.)*

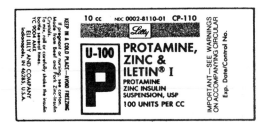 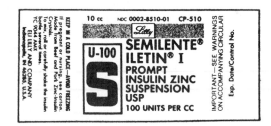

Figure 9-12   *(Courtesy Eli Lilly & Co.)*

taneously or intravenously. It is important to remember that regular insulin is the *only type of insulin* that can be administered intravenously.

Due to the suspension of zinc and/or protamine, modified insulin is cloudy, and *only* can be administered subcutaneously. Figure 9-12 shows two examples.

A combination of regular and modified insulins often will be ordered to provide for both rapid and prolonged action. One such combination, currently on the market, contains 70% modified and 30% regular insulins pre-mixed, Figure 9-13. These insulin mixtures are convenient to use when the prescribed dose is identical to the mixture available. However, in many instances this is not the case. If an identical combination is not available, the ordered insulin dosages may be administered separately or mixed in one syringe for administration. In mixing two different types

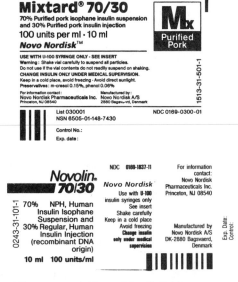

Figure 9-13   *(Courtesy of Novo Nordisk Pharmaceuticals, Inc.)*

of insulin in one syringe, it is important that no modified insulin be introduced into the bottle of regular insulin. Therefore, when mixing two types of insulin in one syringe, the regular insulin (clear) should be drawn up first and the modified insulin (cloudy) second. (See Procedure for Mixing Insulins, page 161.) Because mixtures of insulin remain stable for only a few minutes, it is important to administer these injections immediately after mixing them. Regardless of whether regular, modified, or mixed insulins are ordered, it is essential that the correct type be selected and that the exact prescribed amount be administered.

Insulin preparations should be stored in a cold place, preferably refrigerated, but not frozen. Insulin currently in use may be stored unrefrigerated, as long as it is kept as cool as possible and away from sunlight or direct heat.

Practice: Reading Insulin Labels

From Figure 9-14, select the correct bottle (by letter) and answer the questions relating to the insulin order.

1. What is the concentration of each of the insulin preparations shown?
   _____
2. Identify the two manufacturers represented. _____
3. Select by letter:
   - All of the varieties of human (synthetic) insulin pictured. _____
   - All of the varieties of NPH insulin pictured. _____
   - Two labels identifying insulin modified with both protamine and zinc. _____
   - A regular insulin prepared from beef. _____
   - A semilente insulin prepared from pork. _____
   - All the preparations from a mixed (beef/pork) source. _____
4. What letter appears on the label for:
   - Regular Insulin _____
   - Semilente Insulin _____
   - NPH Insulin _____
   - Lente Insulin _____
   - Ultralente Insulin _____
   - Protamine, Zinc Insulin _____
5. Prepare the following doses of insulin for administration. You have available a 1 cc, U-100 syringe. Select (by letter) the correct medication label from Figure 9-14.
   a. **Order:** Humulin R Insulin 24 U sc
      1. **Label:** _____
      2. How much insulin would you withdraw? _____ U
   b. **Order:** Lente (Pork) Insulin 45 U sc
      1. **Label:** _____
      2. How much insulin would you withdraw? _____ U

TYPES OF INSULIN

FAST-ACTING

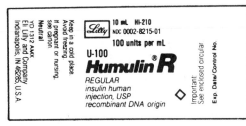

a.

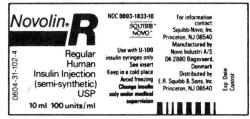

b.

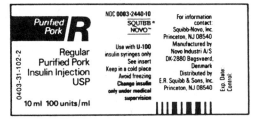

c.

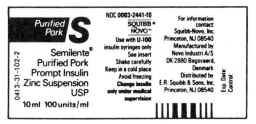

d.

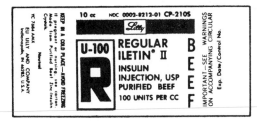

e.

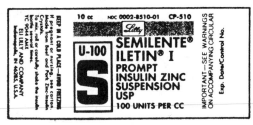

f.

Note: On the Lilly label, Iletin I means the source is mixed beef and pork, Iletin II means the source is pure beef or pure pork.

Figure 9-14　*(Parts a, e, f, g, k, l, o, p, and q Courtesy Eli Lilly & Co.; Parts b, c, d, h, i, j, m, and n Courtesy Squibb-Novo, Inc.)*

INTERMEDIATE

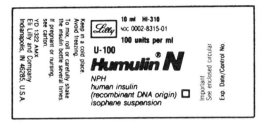

g.

Novolin™ N — NDC 0063-1834-10 — NPH Human Insulin Isophane Suspension (semi-synthetic) — 10 ml 100 units/ml

h.

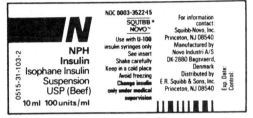

i.

Purified Pork L — NDC 0063-2442-10 — Lente® Purified Pork Insulin Zinc Suspension USP — 10 ml 100 units/ml

j.

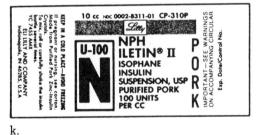

k.

10 cc — NDC 0002-8412-01 — CP-410S — Lilly — U-100 — LENTE® ILETIN® II — INSULIN ZINC SUSPENSION, USP — PURIFIED BEEF — 100 UNITS PER CC — BEEF

l.

LONG-ACTING

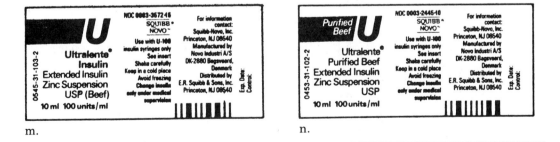

m.

Ultralente® Insulin Extended Insulin Zinc Suspension USP (Beef) — 10 ml 100 units/ml

Purified Beef U — NDC 0063-2445-10 — Ultralente® Purified Beef Extended Insulin Zinc Suspension USP — 10 ml 100 units/ml

n.

Note: On the Lilly label, Iletin I means the source is mixed beef and pork, Iletin II means the source is pure beef or pure pork.

Figure 9-14 Cont.

TYPES OF INSULIN

LONG-ACTING

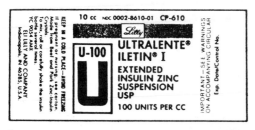

o.

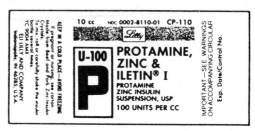

p.

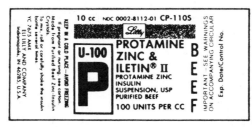

q.

Note: On the Lilly label, Iletin I means the source is mixed beef and pork, Iletin II means the source is pure beef or pure pork.

Figure 9-14   Cont.

c. **Order:** Regular (Beef) Insulin 10 U and Protamine, Zinc (Beef) Insulin 38 U sc
   1. **Labels:** _____
   2. Which insulin would be drawn up first? _____
   3. What is the total amount of insulin mixed in the syringe? _____ U

d. **Order:** Semilente (Purified Pork) Insulin 24 U and Lente (Pork) Insulin 42 U sc
   1. **Labels:** _____
   2. Which insulin would be drawn up last? _____
   3. What is the total amount of insulin mixed in the syringe? _____ U

(*Note:* See Appendix C for answer key.)

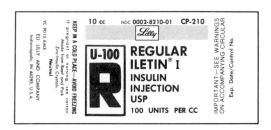

Figure 9-15 *(Courtesy Eli Lilly & Co.)*

Insulin Administration

Insulin is ordered and measured in USP units. Almost universally used is the concentration of 100 units per milliliter, designated on the bottle as U-100 insulin, Figure 9-15. This means that 1 ml of the product contains 100 units of insulin. Insulin syringes for this strength are available in two sizes, a 1 cc size that measures up to 100 units (Figure 9-16) and a 0.5 cc size that measures up to 50 units; these are referred to commonly as U-100 syringes. They usually are pre-packaged with a 27 or 28 gauge, 1/2" needle. Use of the unit-calibrated insulin syringe eliminates the need for calculation, because it is only necessary to draw up the ordered number of units. Neither a tuberculin syringe nor a 2–3 ml syringe gives precise enough measurement; these never should be used for insulin.

Insulin is also available in U-500 concentrations; one ml containing 500 units of insulin. This strength also requires a specially calibrated syringe for measuring. U-500 insulin is a concentration of regular insulin that can be administered by either subcutaneous or intramuscular routes. The intravenous route is not recommended.

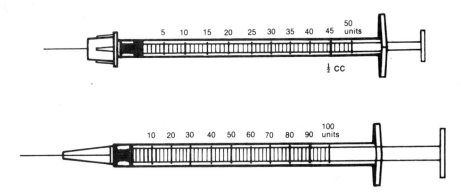

Figure 9-16 Insulin syringes

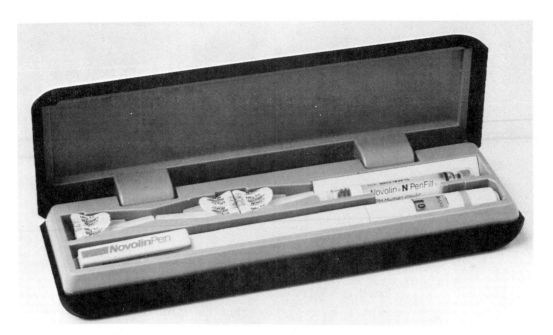

Figure 9-17 Insulin injection system for self-administration *(Courtesy Squibb-Novo, Inc.)*

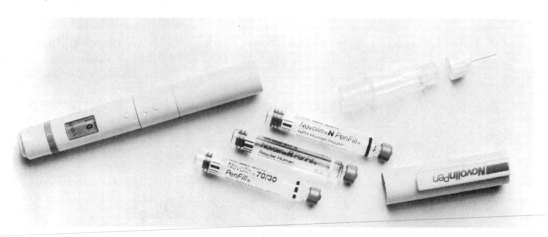

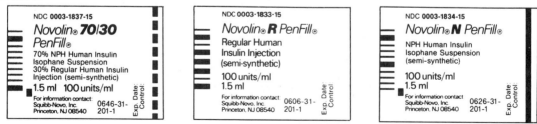

NDC 0003-1837-15

*Novolin® **70/30**
PenFill®*

70% NPH Human Insulin
Isophane Suspension
30% Regular Human Insulin
Injection (semi-synthetic)

1.5 ml   100 units/ml

For information contact:
Squibb-Novo, Inc.   0646-31-
Princeton, NJ 08540   201-1

Exp. Date
Control

NDC 0003-1833-15

*Novolin® **R** PenFill®*

Regular Human
Insulin Injection
(semi-synthetic)

100 units/ml
1.5 ml

For information contact:
Squibb-Novo, Inc.   0606-31-
Princeton, NJ 08540   201-1

Exp. Date
Control

NDC 0003-1834-15

*Novolin® **N** PenFill®*

NPH Human Insulin
Isophane Suspension
(semi-synthetic)

100 units/ml
1.5 ml

For information contact:
Squibb-Novo, Inc.   0626-31-
Princeton, NJ 08540   201-1

Exp. Date
Control

Figure 9-18   *(Courtesy Squibb-Novo, Inc.)*

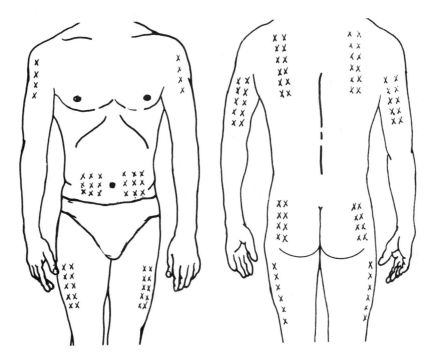

Figure 9-19

It is essential that the calibrations of the syringe match the concentration of the insulin, that is, the number of units per milliliter. The nurse must be careful to ascertain the strength of the insulin being administered and use the correctly calibrated syringe.

Insulin Injection

Because most persons who require insulin injections are eventually taught to self-administer this hormone, nurses must be alert to the learning needs of these patients and must teach and reinforce correct principles of insulin administration.

Because the insulin injection is repeated daily or more often, it is essential to rotate injection sites to prevent tissue damage or complications such as atrophy, thickening, or scarring, all of which can interfere with proper absorption. Patients should be taught to alternate sites using a site selection plan that will help ensure proper rotation.

Patients may also need to learn how to mix combinations of insulin preparations in one syringe. It is important to stress that the short-acting (regular) insulin be withdrawn prior to withdrawal of long-acting (modified) insulin. It is essential that any air bubbles be eliminated from the syringe when obtaining the dose of insulin to have an accurate amount. The step of aspirating for blood prior to injection is omitted in teaching self-administration of insulin, because it is difficult for patients to do this one-handed.

In addition to the insulin syringe and needle, other insulin injection devices are currently available that offer accuracy, convenience, and versatility for persons who self-administer their insulin. One such example, shown in Figure 9-17, can be easily carried about and facilitates daily single or multiple injections of pre-mixed insulin (Figure 9-18), thereby greatly simplifying the procedure and routine of insulin self-administration.

Any area of subcutaneous tissue can be used for insulin administration. Diabetic patients most frequently use the abdomen and thighs for self-administration sites. When insulin is administered by other persons, the upper arms, upper back, and gluteal areas can be used, Figure 9-19.

The following checklist may be used as a guide for insulin administration.

Performance Criteria: Administration of Insulin

(*Note:* Follows usual procedure for subcutaneous injection with the following modifications.)

	S	U	Comments
1. Selects appropriate size (½ or 1 cc) insulin syringe with ½" needle			
2. Rolls vial of modified insulin between hands to mix (avoids shaking)			
*3. When mixing two insulins in one syringe, withdraws regular insulin into syringe first, then modified insulin			
4. Selects correct site according to previously established plan for rotation of sites			
5. Places glove on non-dominant hand			
6. Pinches cleansed site between thumb and forefinger and inserts needle at 90° angle			

Continued on next page

Performance Criteria: Administration of Insulin (Cont.)

(*Note:* Follows usual procedure for subcutaneous injection with the following modifications.)

	S	U	Comments
7. Does not aspirate for blood			
8. Upon withdrawal of needle, places antiseptic wipe over site and presses lightly. Does *NOT* massage			
9. Discards used syringe and needle (without re-capping) into puncture-resistant container			
10. Records administration on diabetic record as well as on medication record and/or site selection plan			

S—Satisfactory   U—Unsatisfactory   Evaluator _____

*Procedure for Mixing Insulins (clear to cloudy)
1. Obtain correct insulin vials and correct insulin syringe/needle
2. Cleanse top of modified (cloudy) insulin and inject air into air space equal to desired dose
3. Cleanse top of regular (clear) insulin and inject air into air space equal to desired dose, then withdraw desired dose of regular insulin
4. Insert needle into vial of modified insulin and withdraw desired dose, being careful not to introduce any regular insulin into vial
5. Gently rotate syringe to mix insulins

Calculations of Intravenous Medications and Solutions

••

Objectives

Upon completion of this unit of study you should be able to:
- *Identify equipment used in the administration of intravenous medications and solutions, including types of needles and cannulas, infusion sets, and solution containers.*
- *Describe the various methods by which intravenous medications/solutions may be administered: continuous IV drip, IV piggyback, volume control set, heparin lock, central venous catheter, and IV bolus.*
- *Read drug labels to obtain necessary information for administration of IV medications and solutions.*
- *Demonstrate knowledge of the appropriate method for rounding off when calculating IV flow rates.*
- *Apply the label factor method to clinical calculations involving medications administered intravenously.*
- *Identify nursing responsibilities in relation to assessing and adjusting intravenous infusions.*

Intravenous Injections and Infusions

Intravenous administration refers to the injection or infusion of medications and fluids into a vein. It is another example of parenteral administration. Because the medication enters the circulation directly, the effect of drugs given intravenously is immediate. The abbreviation IV is used for these medication orders.

This unit deals with equipment and solutions used in administering IVs, reading labels and adding medications, and calculating IV drug dosages.

Equipment

Needles, Catheters, and Cannulas

Generally, a needle with a plastic catheter attached is used to administer intravenous fluids. After venipuncture, the cathether is threaded into the vein and remains in place when the needle is withdrawn. This combination needle/catheter is called a cannula. A plastic catheter that passes through the needle bore (inside-the-needle catheter) is called an intracath; one that covers the needle (over-the-needle catheter) is called an angiocath. Intravenous catheters vary in length from 1¼ to 36″ and in diameter from 12G to 22G, and they are used when prolonged infusions are administered.

Large gauge (18 or 19) needles or catheters are used for administering blood or viscous liquids such as hyperalimentation fluid. For venipunctures on infants and children or for adults with small veins, a wing tip (butterfly) needle of suitable length may be used. On infants, a scalp vein butterfly needle may be preferable, Figure 10-1A.

Needleless IV devices that greatly reduce the risk of IV contamination via air, blood, or touch, and also reduce the risk of accidental needle-stick injuries are currently available Figure 10-1B, 10-1C.

Infusion Sets

There is a variety of IV administration sets available for use as primary setups for continuous infusion and secondary setups for intermittent infu-

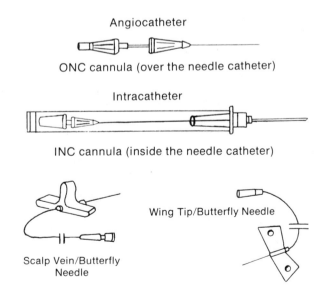

Figure 10-1A   Needles and cannulas used for IVs

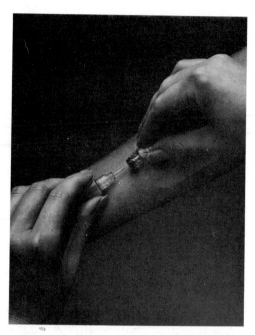

Figure 10-1B The InterLink™ IV Access System requires minimal change in technique (*InterLink™ is a trademark of Baxter Healthcare Corp.*)

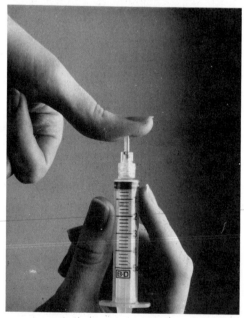

Figure 10-1B Cont. The InterLink™ IV Access System syringe cannula replaces the conventional needle, thus eliminating the risk of accidental needlesticks (*InterLink™ is a trademark of Baxter Healthcare Corp.*)

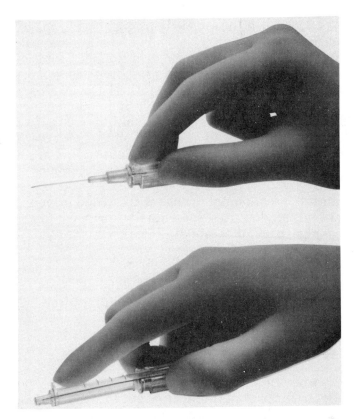

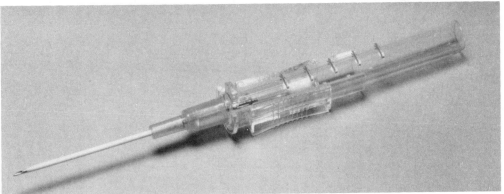

Figure 10-1C   The PROTECTIV™ IV Catheter Safety System has built-in needlestick protection. As the user slides the catheter off the introducer needle, a protective guard glides over the contaminated needle before it is removed from the catheter hub. A reassuring "click" tells the user when the needle is locked safely inside the guard (*Courtesy Critikon, Inc.*)

sion. All sets consist of intravenous tubing, some type of drip chamber, a regulator clamp, and protective caps to maintain sterility.

The size of the opening into the drip chamber determines the size of the drop delivered by the infusion set. The most common sizes (called macrodrip) are calibrated to deliver 10, 15, or 20 drops per milliliter. Microdrip (minidrip) sets, calibrated to administer small and very precise amounts of fluid, deliver 60 drops per milliliter, Figure 10–2. The drop size, called the *drop factor*, is identified on the package. The drop factor refers to the number of drops needed to deliver 1 ml of fluid, and always should be determined prior to calculating and/or adjusting the flow rate, Figure 10-3.

Infusion sets are adapted for use with vented or non-vented solution containers and may be used individually (primary line) or attached to each other (piggyback or secondary lines).

Reading Labels: Drop Factor

From Figure 10-4, answer the following questions:

1. What is the calibration in drops per milliliter (drop factor) for each of the infusion sets?
    a. _____
    b. _____
    c. _____
2. Which is/are macrodrip set(s)? _____
3. Which is/are microdrip (minidrip) set(s)? _____

(*Note:* See Appendix C for answer key.)

IV Drops

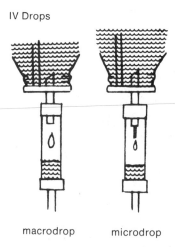

macrodrop   microdrop

Figure 10-2

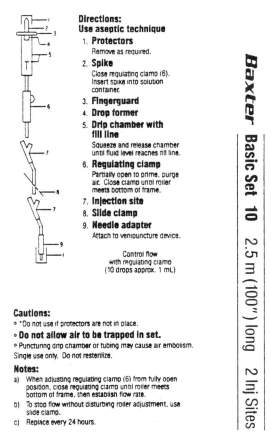

Directions:
Use aseptic technique

1. **Protectors**
   Remove as required.

2. **Spike**
   Close regulating clamp (6).
   Insert spike into solution
   container.

3. **Fingerguard**

4. **Drop former**

5. **Drip chamber with**
   fill line
   Squeeze and release chamber
   until fluid level reaches fill line.

6. **Regulating clamp**
   Partially open to prime, purge
   air. Close clamp until roller
   meets bottom of frame.

7. **Injection site**

8. **Slide clamp**

9. **Needle adapter**
   Attach to venipuncture device.

Control flow
with regulating clamp
(10 drops approx. 1 mL)

Baxter Basic Set 10   2.5 m (100") long   2 Inj Sites

Cautions:

○ *Do not use if protectors are not in place.

○ **Do not allow air to be trapped in set.**

○ Puncturing drip chamber or tubing may cause air embolism.
Single use only. Do not resterilize.

Notes:

a) When adjusting regulating clamp (6) from fully open
   position, close regulating clamp until roller meets
   bottom of frame, then establish flow rate.

b) To stop flow without disturbing roller adjustment, use
   slide clamp.

c) Replace every 24 hours.

Figure 10-3 *(Supplied by Baxter Healthcare Corporation, Deerfield, Illinois 60015 USA.* **Note: This product labeling is a sample and is subject to change at any time. Be sure to read the directions for use accompanying the product.)**

Intravenous Solution Containers

Intravenous solution containers are made of glass or plastic and come in a variety of sizes and shapes. Glass containers are vacuum sealed and have rubber stoppers with openings for the tubing, for venting, and/or for the addition of medications. Plastic containers have special ports for insertion of tubing and addition of medications. All containers are calibrated according to the amount of fluid contained and are labeled as to type of solution, instructions for use, and other pertinent information.

a.

10 drops approx. 1 mL
2.5 m (100″) long

Caution: Federal (USA) law restricts this device
to sale by or on order of a physician.

2C5425 s

Baxter
Basic Set
10

b.

Nitroglycerin   No. 1772
Primary I.V. Set-SL
Vented, 107 Inch

15
DROPS/mL

c.

Nitroglycerin MICRODRIP® No. 9252
IV Micro Pump Set-SL
Vented, 107 Inch

60
DROPS/mL
TYPE A

Figure 10-4 (*Part a supplied by Baxter Healthcare Corporation, Deerfield, Illinois 60015 USA.* **Note: This product labeling is a sample and is subject to change at any time. Be sure to read the directions for use accompanying the product.** *Parts b and c Courtesy Abbott Laboratories*)

Reading IV Labels

Figure 10-5

1. What is the total amount of solution in the container? _____
2. What percentage of the solution is dextrose? _____
3. What is the name of the manufacturer? _____

Figure 10-6

1. What is the total amount of solution in the container? _____
2. What percentage of the solution is Sodium Chloride?* _____
   *This percentage solution is also called Normal Saline and orders may be written using the abbreviation NS.

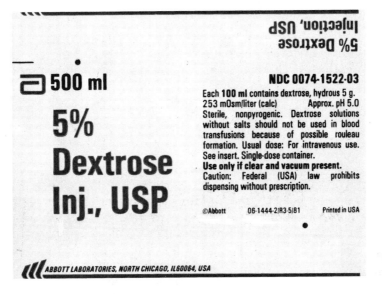

Figure 10-5 (*Courtesy Abbott Laboratories*)

250 ml
0.9% Sodium Chloride
Inj., USP

Figure 10-6 (*Courtesy Abbott Laboratories*)

1000 ml
5% DEXTROSE AND LACTATED RINGER'S
INJECTION, USP
Each 100 ml contains 600 mg
Sodium Chloride USP, 310 mg
Sodium Lactate, 30 mg Potassium
Chloride USP, 20 mg Calcium
Chloride USP

Figure 10-7 (*Courtesy Abbott Laboratories*)

Figure 10-7
1. What is the total amount of solution in the container? _____
2. What percentage of the solution is dextrose? _____
3. What other chemical ingredients does the solution contain? _____
(*Note:* See Appendix C for answer key.)

Intermittent IV Drug Administration

IV Piggyback (IVPB)

Medications often are given intravenously by adding a secondary infusion line to an existing IV line. This is called the piggyback method and often is used to administer medications that are ordered at regularly scheduled times (i.e., intermittent drug administration) (e.g., q 6 hr).

Medications administered via piggyback usually are diluted in 50–100 ml of solution. They may be infused simultaneously or alternately with a primary infusion. The piggyback set includes a small IV bottle or bag, a drip chamber, short tubing, and a needle (usually 20 gauge, 1″) that is inserted into the primary line through a special port, Figure 10-8.

Volume Control Set

This is a special infusion set designed to administer small amounts of fluid over a specified time period, usually 30–60 minutes. It consists of a small fluid chamber, drip chamber, and tubing, and can be used as either a primary or secondary infusion line, Figure 10-9. The fluid chamber holds 100 ml or more, to which medications can be added through a medication port. The drip chamber is calibrated at 60 gtt/ml (micro- or minidrip) and the IV flow rate is regulated by adjusting the clamp below this chamber. These sets often are referred to by their brand names such as *Buretrol, Volutrol,* and *Metriset.*

Saline Lock

The saline lock, also called saline well, is a device that serves as an intermittent IV line. It may be used for administration of regularly scheduled IV medications for patients who do not also require parenteral fluids, thus eliminating the need for a continuous IV. Alternatively, a saline lock may be inserted for the purpose of administering IV medications that are incompatible with solutions or drugs concurrently being given IV.

The device consists of an IV needle or catheter attached to a short plastic tube that terminates in a rubber seal, Figure 10-10. Medication is injected or infused through the seal at the designated times. Because the needle or catheter remains in the vein, it must be flushed periodically with saline to prevent clot formation and to maintain patency. In some

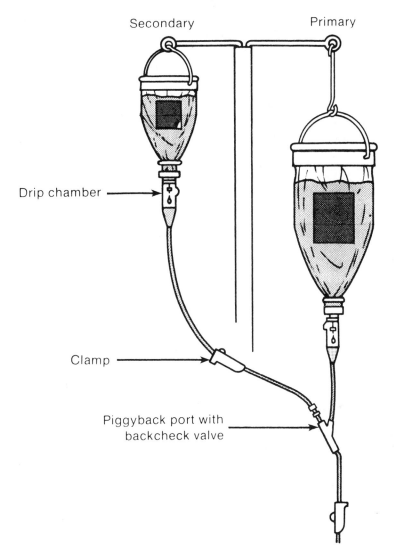

Figure 10-8 IV piggyback

instances, depending on hospital policy, diluted heparin is injected following the saline flush. (The saline lock sometimes is referred to as the heparin lock.)

Central Venous Catheter

Medications can be infused through a catheter that is inserted into a major vein and usually advanced from this vein into the superior vena

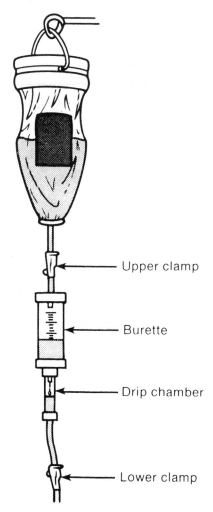

Upper clamp

Burette

Drip chamber

Lower clamp

Figure 10-9   IV volume control set

cava. If the catheter also is to be used for measuring central venous pressure, it is directed through the vena cava into the right atrium. Because the catheter is left in place, it can be used for a continuous or intermittent infusion line. Veins most commonly used for central venous lines are the subclavian and the external jugular, although the brachial and femoral veins are alternative routes.

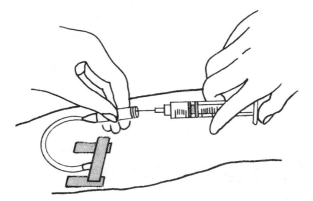

Figure 10-10 Saline lock

A very useful modification of the central venous catheter is a multilumen catheter that permits a variety of treatment and monitoring procedures to be performed via a single venipuncture site.

One such device is pictured in Figure 10-11. This catheter, which contains three lumens, can be used in place of multiple central and peripheral lines for patients who require a multiplicity of intravenous therapy and monitoring, often several procedures simultaneously. This versatile central venous catheter provides routes for fluid administration, TPN (total parenteral nutrition), blood sampling, central venous pressure monitoring, and medication administration, including simultaneous infusion of incompatible drugs.

The multi-lumen catheter must be flushed periodically with saline to maintain patency of lumens that are used intermittently. The procedure is similar to that used with the saline lock. A lumen that is being used for a continuous IV infusion does not need to be flushed.

Intravenous Regulators

Intravenous regulators are electronic pumps and controllers that help provide accuracy and safety in administration of IV therapy. Controllers automatically regulate the drop rate of infusions where the force of gravity provides the needed pressure to maintain fluid flow, Figure 10-12.

Pumps fall into two categories, the IV regulator pump and the syringe pump. The IV regulator pump maintains fluid flow by means of positive pressure, which can be varied or adjusted as needed, Figure 10-13. The syringe pump, also called a mini-infuser, is used when a small amount of medication (e.g., up to 60 ml) is administered. The medication is infused from a syringe that is inserted into the apparatus, Figure 10-14.

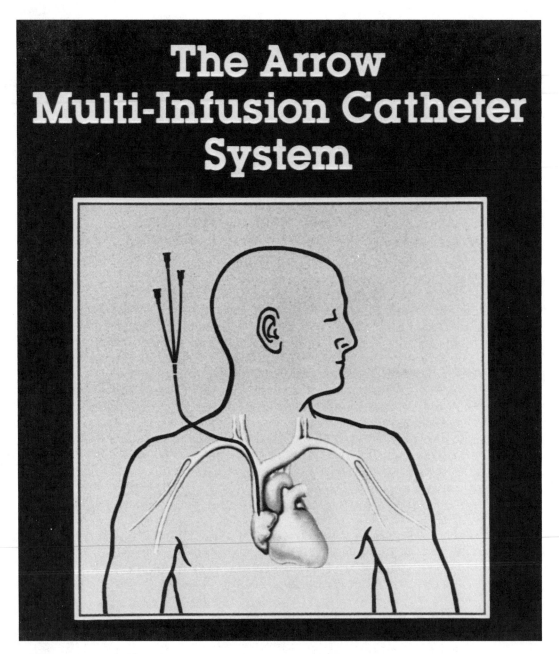

Figure 10-11   Multi-lumen central venous catheter for CVP monitoring and/or multiple infusions at one puncture site (*Courtesy Arrow International, Inc.*)

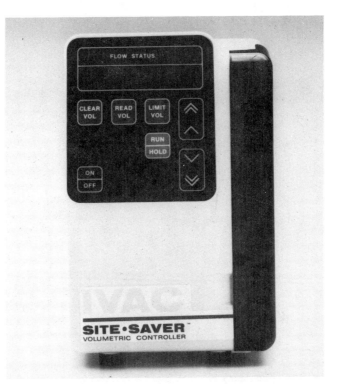

Figure 10-12 Volumetric controller (*Courtesy IVAC Corporation*)

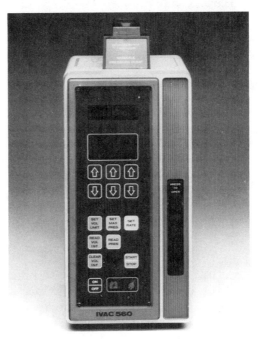

Figure 10-13 Variable pressure pump (*Courtesy IVAC Corporation*)

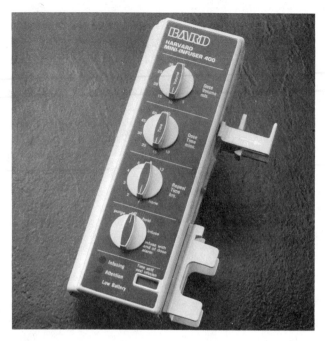

Figure 10-14 Harvard mini-infuser (*Courtesy Bard® Med Systems Division*)

Pumps and controllers have a variety of mechanisms for automatically regulating drop rate and/or fluid volume and for providing warning alarms when there is a problem with the infusion or equipment.

Calculation of Intravenous Flow Rates, Infusion Times, Infusion Rate, and Bolus Using Label Factor Method

Once the infusion is started, the nurse is responsible for regulating the flow rate (i.e., the number of drops per minute required to infuse the IV within the time period or infusion rate specified).

In calculating the flow rate for *drops per minute,* one minute becomes the labeled value that must be converted to an equivalent value: number of drops. *One minute,* therefore, is the starting factor and *drops* is the answer label and these, as in all label factor conversions, form an equivalent relationship.

It is essential in calculating flow rate to know the drop factor. This refers to the size of the drop delivered by the particular infusion set being used: the number of drops required to make 1 ml (cc). The drop factor always will be stated in practice problems requiring calculation of drops per minute.

Rounding Off

The rate of flow should be rounded to the nearest whole number.

1. 31.6 gtt/min; adjust to 32 gtt/min
2. 42.3 gtt/min; adjust to 42 gtt/min
3. 56.8 ml/hr; adjust to 57 ml/hr
4. 120.4 ml/hr; adjust to 120 ml/hr

Calculation of IV Flow Rate When Total Infusion Time is Specified

Example:

Order: 1000 ml of D5W (5% Dextrose in water) IV to infuse over a period of 5 hr

Drop Factor: 10 gtt/ml

Equivalents: 1000 ml = 5 hr, 10 gtt = 1 ml, 60 min = 1 hr

Conversion Equation: $1 \text{ min} \times \dfrac{1 \text{ hr}}{60 \text{ min}} \times \dfrac{1000 \text{ ml}}{5 \text{ hr}} \times \dfrac{10 \text{ gtt}}{1 \text{ ml}} = 33.3 = 33 \text{ gtt}$

Flow Rate: 33 gtt/min

Calculation of IV Flow Rate When an Infusion Rate is Specified

Examples:

a. **Order:** 1500 ml of Sodium Chloride 0.9% (0.9% Sodium Chloride Solution) to infuse at a rate of 90 ml/hr

Drop Factor: 20 gtt/ml

Starting Factor   Answer Label
    1 min   gtt

Equivalents: 90 ml = 1 hr, 20 gtt = 1 ml, 60 min = 1 hr

Conversion Equation: $1 \text{ min} \times \dfrac{1 \text{ hr}}{60 \text{ min}} \times \dfrac{90 \text{ ml}}{1 \text{ hr}} \times \dfrac{20 \text{ gtt}}{1 \text{ ml}} = 30 \text{ gtt}$

Flow Rate: 30 gtt/min

b. **Order:** 1000 ml of 5% D ½ NSS (5% Dextrose in ½ Normal Saline Solution) to infuse at a rate of 100 ml/hr

Drop Factor: 60 gtt/ml

Starting Factor   Answer Label
    1 min   gtt

Equivalents: 100 ml = 1 hr, 60 gtt = 1 ml, 60 min = 1 hr

Conversion Equation: $1 \text{ min} \times \dfrac{1 \text{ hr}}{60 \text{ min}} \times \dfrac{100 \text{ ml}}{1 \text{ hr}} \times \dfrac{60 \text{ gtt}}{1 \text{ ml}} = 100 \text{ gtt}$

*Flow rate: 100 gtt/min

> **Note:* When using any infusion set having a drop factor of 60 gtt/ml (sometimes written as: drop factor microdrip), the flow rate per minute *always* will be the same as the number of ml per hour. For example:
>
> Order: 50 ml/hr; flow rate: 50 gtt/min
> Order: 70 ml/hr; flow rate: 70 gtt/min
>
> Therefore, the flow rate calculation can be omitted for this type of order.

c. **Order:** 500 ml D5W IV KVO

The abbreviation KVO stands for Keep Vein Open (or TKO = To Keep Open). This means that the IV is to run at a very slow rate simply to have an infusion route available for emergency use or intermittent administration of drugs. A microdrip infusion set usually is used. A typical flow rate, which may vary according to hospital policy, is 10–20 ml/hr.

It can be seen from the box above that no calculation is necessary for a KVO order, because the flow rate will be the same as the stated ml/hr; in this case, 10–20 gtt/min.

Practice: Calculation of IV Flow Rate When Total Infusion Time Is Specified

1. **Order:** 1500 ml of D5W IV to infuse in 8 hr
   Drop Factor: 10 gtt/ml

2. **Order:** 1000 ml NS to infuse in 10 hr
   Drop Factor: 15 gtt/ml

3. **Order:** 800 ml 5% glucose in water in 4 hr
   Drop Factor: 15 gtt/ml

4. **Order:** 700 ml D5W IV in 5 hr
   Drop Factor: 10 gtt/ml

5. **Order:** 2500 ml 5% Dextrose in 0.45 NS IV in 24 hr
   Drop Factor: 20 gtt/ml

6. **Order:** 1250 ml D 2.5 W IV in 6 hr
   Drop Factor: 15 gtt/ml

7. **Order:** 500 ml Sodium Chloride 0.9% IV in 3 hr
   Drop Factor: 10 gtt/ml

8. **Order:** 100 ml Ringers IV in 4 hr
   Drop Factor: 15 gtt/ml

9. **Order:** 300 ml D5W IV in 3 hr
   Drop Factor: 60 gtt/ml

10. **Order:** 50 cc Serum Albumin IV to infuse in 1 hr
    Drop Factor: 15 gtt/ml

Practice: Calculation of IV Flow Rate When an Infusion Rate Is Specified

11. **Order:** 1000 ml Ringers IV to infuse at a rate of 125 ml/hr
    Drop Factor: 15 gtt/ml
    What should the flow rate be per minute?

12. **Order:** 1000 ml D5W IV to infuse at a rate of 100 ml/hr
    Drop Factor: 10 gtt/ml
    What should the flow rate be per minute?

13. **Order:** 1500 ml Sodium Chloride 0.9% IV to infuse at a rate of 150 ml/hr
   Drop Factor: 15 gtt/ml
   What should the flow rate be per minute?

14. **Order:** 2000 ml of D2.5W IV to infuse at a rate of 125 ml/hr
   Drop Factor: 10 gtt/ml
   What should the flow rate be per minute?

15. **Order:** 500 ml Isolyte M IV to infuse at a rate of 125 ml/hr
   Drop Factor: 60 gtt/ml
   What should the flow rate be per minute?

16. **Order:** Hyperalimentation (TPN) 1000 ml D20W IV to infuse at a rate of 80 ml/hr
   Drop Factor: 15 gtt/ml
   What should the flow rate be per minute?

17. **Order:** Hyperalimentation (TPN) 1000 ml Aminosyn 3.5% IV to in-
fuse at a rate of 40 ml/hr
Drop Factor: 20 gtt/ml
What should the flow rate be per minute?

(*Note:* See Appendix C for answer key.)

Calculation of Flow Rate (GTT/MIN) When IV Contains Medication

The IV flow rate is calculated the same whether or not medication has
been added to the IV container. If medication is to be added, however,
the additional numbers in the order may cause confusion in determining
the conversion factors. It is, therefore, essential to carefully inspect the
information given and select the correct equivalents for the conversion
equation.

Example:

Order: Ampicillin 500 mg in 50 ml of Sodium Chloride 0.9% to infuse
in 1 hr.

Drop Factor: 60 gtt/ml

Starting Factor   Answer Label
    1 min   gtt

Equivalents: 50 ml = 1 hr, 60 gtt = 1 ml, 60 min = 1 hr

Conversion Equation: $1 \, \cancel{\text{min}} \times \dfrac{1 \, \cancel{\text{hr}}}{60 \, \cancel{\text{min}}} \times \dfrac{50 \, \cancel{\text{ml}}}{1 \, \cancel{\text{hr}}} \times \dfrac{60 \, \text{gtt}}{1 \, \cancel{\text{ml}}} = 50 \, \text{gtt}$

Flow Rate: 50 gtt/min

(*Note:* the medication (Ampicillin 500 mg) that is added to the total
amount of IV solution (50 ml) and the 0.9% NaCl are not pertinent to the
computation of the flow rate and are not included in the conversion
equation.)

Practice: Calculation of Flow Rate When IV Contains Medication

1. **Order:** 1000 ml D5NS with KCl 40 mEq IV to infuse in 4 hr
Drop Factor: 15 gtt/ml

2. **Order:** 250 ml D5W with Aminophylline 0.5 Gm IV to infuse in 2 hr
   Drop Factor: 60 gtt/ml

3. **Order:** Geopen (carbenicillin disodium) 2 Gm in 50 ml Sodium Chloride 0.9% to infuse in 30 min
   Drop Factor: 15 gtt/ml

4. **Order:** Erythromycin 500 mg in 100 ml D5W to infuse in 20 min
   Drop Factor: 10 gtt/ml

5. **Order:** Cleocin (clindamycin) 600 mg in 100 ml D5W to infuse in 60 min
   Drop Factor: 20 gtt/ml

(*Note:* See Appendix C for answer key.)

Calculation of IV Flow Rate When an Infusion Pump is Used

Intravenous (infusion) pumps are useful, because they maintain a more accurate flow rate than is possible with the standard IV (gravity) administration set. The most commonly used pumps are: volumetric and nonvolumetric.

Nonvolumetric pumps are designed to administer a certain number of drops per minute. The flow rate is determined in gtt/min and the pump is set to deliver this amount. Nonvolumetric pumps have been replaced by volumetric systems for the most part.

Volumetric pumps are designed to administer fluid in milliliters per hour. The flow rate is determined in ml/hr and the corresponding gtt/min rate is determined from a conversion chart that usually is printed on the infusion apparatus.

Example:

Order: 500 ml D5½NS IV to infuse at a 10 hr rate (i.e., over a period of 10 hr). Use an infusion pump.

How many ml/hr should be administered?

Starting Factor   Answer Label
     1 hr   ml

Equivalents: 500 ml = 10 hr

Conversion Equation: $1 \, hr \times \dfrac{500 \, ml}{10 \, hr} = 50 \, ml$

The number of *drops per minute* required to deliver this amount of *solution per hour* depends on the drop factor of the tubing being used (e.g., 10-15-20-60 gtt/ml). In this case, because an infusion pump is being used, the drops per minute would be determined by consulting the operating manual or a conversion chart on the pump, Table 10-1.

Find the drops/min setting for the above flow rate (50 ml/hr). The infusion set has a tubing drop factor of 20 gtt/ml.

Answer: The pump would be set to deliver 17 gtt/min.

Practice: Calculation of the Number of ml/hr That Will Infuse

1. **Order:** 1000 ml 5% D/NS IV to infuse at an 8 hr rate

2. **Order:** 500 ml Lactated Ringers IV to infuse at a 6 hr rate

Table 10-1.   CONVERSION BETWEEN ML/HR AND GTT/MIN

DESIRED RATE ML/HR	GTT/MIN SETTING			
	Tubing Drop Factor			
	10	15	20	60
10	2	3	3	10
20	3	5	7	20
30	5	8	10	30
40	7	10	13	40
50	8	13	(17)	50
60	10	15	20	60

3. **Order:** 1500 ml 2.5% D 0.45 NaCl IV to infuse at a 12 hr rate

4. **Order:** 250 ml D 2.5/W IV to infuse at a 2 hr rate

5. **Order:** 2500 ml NS IV to infuse at a 24 hr rate

6. **Order:** Hyperalimentation (TPN) 2000 ml Liposyn II 20% IV to infuse in 24 hr

7. **Order:** Hyperalimentation (TPN) 3000 ml Aminosyn 8.5% IV to infuse in 24 hr

(*Note:* See Appendix C for answer key.)

Calculation of Infusion Time

The label factor method can be used to calculate the anticipated length of time required for an infusion to be completed. (*Note:* When doing these problems, carry answers to hundredths and round to tenths. Convert to hr or min.)

Example:

Order: 1500 ml D2.5W IV
Drop Factor: 15 gtt/ml
Flow Rate: 40 gtt/min
How many hours will it take for the IV to infuse?

In this problem, the value sought is the length of time required to infuse a certain amount. The unit of time, therefore, becomes the answer label. The quantity that will be converted to a unit of time (1500 ml) becomes the starting factor. The conversion equation is set up and solved in the usual manner.

Starting Factor   Answer Label
   1500 ml   hours
Equivalents: 15 gtt = 1 ml, 40 gtt = 1 min, 60 min = 1 hr

Conversion Equation: $1500 \, \text{ml} \times \dfrac{15 \, \text{gtt}}{1 \, \text{ml}} \times \dfrac{1 \, \text{min}}{40 \, \text{gtt}} \times \dfrac{1 \, \text{hr}}{60 \, \text{min}} = 9.4$

$$= 9 \, \text{hr} \, 24 \, \text{min}^*$$

*Convert the decimal to minutes by multiplying by 60.

Practice: Calculation of Infusion Time

1. **Order:** 1500 ml Lactated Ringers IV
   Drop Factor: 10 gtt/ml
   Flow Rate: 20 gtt/min
   How long should it take the IV to infuse?

2. **Order:** 750 ml D10W IV
   Drop Factor: 15 gtt/ml
   Flow Rate: 21 gtt/min
   How long should it take the IV to infuse?

3. **Order:** 500 ml of Sodium Chloride 0.9% IV
   Drop Factor: 60 gtt/ml
   Flow Rate: 125 gtt/min
   How long should it take the IV to infuse?

4. **Order:** 2000 ml D5W
   Drop Factor: 15 gtt/ml
   Flow Rate: 34 gtt/min
   How long should it take the IV to infuse?

5. **Order:** 1000 ml D2.5NS IV
   Drop Factor: 10 gtt/ml
   Flow Rate: 23 gtt/min
   How long should it take the IV to infuse?

(*Note:* See Appendix C for answer key.)

Adding Medications to Intravenous Fluids

Intravenous medications can be administered in several ways. They may be added directly to a traditional IV set up, called a primary line, for continuous drip. For intermittent doses (e.g., every 8 or 12 hours), medications may be added to a second line that is then connected to the primary line, or they may be infused through a central venous line. Medications also can be injected directly into a vein (IV bolus) using a syringe and needle; through a primary line via the flashball or a Y-port; or through a saline lock. The medication order should state clearly the desired IV route of administration.

If two or more medications are added to the same IV, it is essential that the substances be compatible. The person mixing and adding substances to an IV has responsibility for ascertaining compatibility. Information about drug compatibility is obtained from the pharmacist, a drug reference book, the manufacturer's product insert, or a drug incompatibility chart.

Whenever a substance is added to an IV, the container must be labeled with the name, dosage, date, and time added.

Medications that are dispensed in liquid form may be added to the IV container through a medication port for infusion or through the tubing or saline lock for injection. Medications that are dispensed as dry powders or crystals must be reconstituted just prior to infusion or injection. Instructions for reconstitution are printed in the package insert or on the medication label. Reconstitution and mixing of intravenous medications usually is done by a registered pharmacist in a controlled area (e.g., under laminar air flow hood) in the pharmacy. Nurses may add medication to existing infusions, but rarely reconstitute.

Remember that only solvents designated in the directions should be used for reconstitution, because these have been determined to be compatible with this particular drug. In addition, when reconstituted drugs are added to IV solutions, it is likewise essential that drug and solution are compatible.

Depending on the amount (volume) of drug that is added to an IV, the total amount of solution to be administered may need to be adjusted in writing the conversion equation for determining flow rate. Several methods may be used. The practitioner may choose the method most appropriate to the situation.

    a. If the amount (volume) of drug to be added is 5% or more of the total amount ordered to be administered, add the two amounts together in the conversion equation.

    b. If the amount (volume) of drug to be added is less than 5% of the total amount ordered to be administered, this amount usually is considered negligible and it is not necessary to add the two amounts together in the conversion equation.

   c. Remove from the IV container an amount of solution sufficient to reconstitute a powdered drug, then return the reconstituted solution to the container, thus not significantly changing the ordered quantity to be administered.

   d. Remove from the IV container and discard an amount of solution equal to that which will be replaced by the ordered amount (volume) of drug. This approach is especially desirable in situations where fluid intake is strictly limited and/or measured.

Adding Drugs to IVs and Calculating Flow Rate in gtt/min

Examples:

1. **Order:** Vibramycin 75 mg in 1000 ml Normosol-M in D5W IV to run in 24 hr

   Label: Vibramycin (doxycycline hyclate) 100 mg (Figure 10-15)

   Directions for reconstitution: Add 10 ml sterile water for injection to yield a concentration of 10 mg/ml.

   a. How much of the reconstituted solution must be added to the IV bottle to provide the ordered dose of Vibramycin 150 mg?

      Equivalent: 10 mg = 1 ml

$$\text{Conversion Equation: } 75\ \cancel{mg} \times \frac{1\ ml}{10\ \cancel{mg}} = 7.5\ ml$$

      Add Vibramycin 7.5 ml to 1000 ml Normosol-M in D5W.

   b. What should the flow rate be for this IV order?

      Drop Factor: 15 gtt/ml

      Equivalents: 1000 ml = 24 hr, 60 min = 1 hr, 15 gtt = 1 ml

$$\text{Conversion Equation: } 1\ \cancel{min} \times \frac{1\ \cancel{hr}}{60\ \cancel{min}} \times \frac{1000\ \cancel{ml}}{24\ \cancel{hr}} \times \frac{15\ gtt}{1\ \cancel{ml}} = 10.4$$
$$= 10\ gtt$$

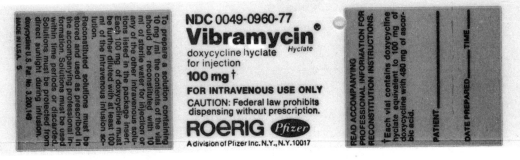

Figure 10-15 (*Courtesy Roerig, A Division of Pfizer Inc.*)

Note: Because the 7.5 ml of reconstituted drug is less than 5% of the total volume (1000 ml) ordered to be administered, it is not necessary to add these amounts together in the conversion equation.

2. **Order:** Ticar 3 Gm in 100 ml Lactated Ringers IV to run in 2 hr
   Label: Ticar (ticarcillin disodium) 3 Gm
   Directions for reconstituting: Add 12 ml sterile water for injection to yield a concentration of 200 mg/ml.
   a. How much of the reconstituted solution must be added to the IV bottle to provide the ordered dose of Ticar 3 Gm?
   Equivalents: 1 Gm = 1000 mg   200 mg = 1 ml

   Conversion Equation: $3 \, \text{Gm} \times \dfrac{1000 \, \text{mg}}{1 \, \text{Gm}} \times \dfrac{1 \, \text{ml}}{200 \, \text{mg}} = 15 \, \text{ml}$
   Add Ticar 15 ml to 100 ml Lactated Ringers Solution
   b. What should the flow rate be for this IV order?
   Drop Factor: 60 gtt/ml
   Equivalents: 1 hr = 60 min   115 ml = 2 hr   60 gtt = 1 ml

   Conversion Equation:

   $1 \, \text{min} \times \dfrac{1 \, \text{hr}}{60 \, \text{min}} \times \dfrac{115 \, \text{ml}}{2 \, \text{hr}} \times \dfrac{60 \, \text{gtt}}{1 \, \text{ml}} = 57.5 = 58 \, \text{gtt}$

Note: Because the 15 ml of reconstituted drug is greater than 5% of the total volume (100 ml) ordered to be administered, it is necessary to add these amounts together in the conversion equation.

Practice: Adding Drugs to IVs and Calculating Flow Rate in gtt/min

1. **Order:** Kefzol 350 mg in 100 ml 5% D/LR IV to run in 60 min.
   Label: Figure 10-16. What is the generic name? _____
   Drop Factor: 15 gtt/ml
   a. How much diluent must be added to the vial to reconstitute the drug for intravenous use?

   b. How much of the resulting solution must be added to the IV bottle to provide the ordered dose of Kefzol 350 mg?

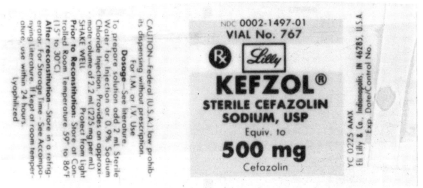

Figure 10-16   (*Courtesy Eli Lilly & Co.*)

c. What should the flow rate be for this IV order?

2. **Order:** Folic Acid 12 mg in 500 ml D5W in 4 hours
   Label: Figure 10-17
   Drop Factor: 60 gtt/ml
   a. How many ml of Folvite must be added to the IV bottle to provide
   the ordered dose?

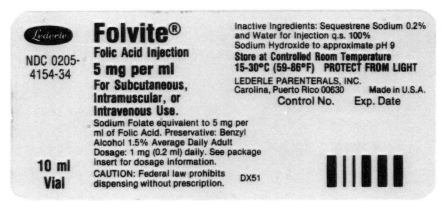

Figure 10-17   (*Courtesy Lederle Laboratories*)

b. What should the flow rate be for this IV order?

3. **Order:** Ampicillin Sodium 150 mg in 1000 ml M/6 Sodium Lactate
   IV to infuse at a rate of 150 ml/hr
   Label: Figure 10-18. What is the trade name? _____
   Drop Factor: 15 gtt/ml
   a. How many ml of Ampicillin Sodium must be added to the IV bottle
   to provide the total ordered dose?

b. What should the flow rate be to administer the ordered number
   of ml/hr?

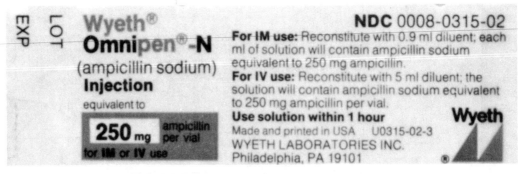

Figure 10-18 *(Courtesy Wyeth Laboratories)*

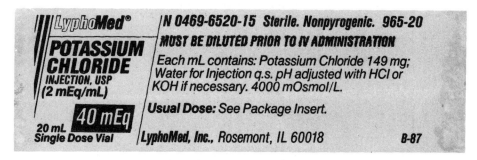

Figure 10-19   (*Courtesy LyphoMed, Inc.*)

4. **Order:** Potassium Chloride (KCl) 30 mEq in 1000 ml D5NS IV in 6 hr
   Label: Potassium Chloride (KCl) injection 40 mEq in 20 ml vial,
   Figure 10-19

(*Note:* This medication is already in solution; therefore, reconstitution
is not necessary.)

   Drop Factor: 10 gtt/ml
   a. How many ml of this medication must be added to the IV bottle
      to provide the ordered dose of KCl 30 mEq?

   b. What should the flow rate be for this IV order?

5. **Order:** Tetracycline 150 mg in 100 ml Sodium Chloride 0.9% to
            infuse in 40 min via Volutrol
   Label: Tetracycline 250 mg
   Directions: Dilute with 5 ml sterile water for injection and add to
            ordered IV solution.
   Drop Factor: 60 gtt/ml

a. How many ml of the reconstituted solution should be added to the IV solution?

b. What should the flow rate be for this IV order?

6. **Order:** Cefoxitin Sodium 2 Gm IV in 100 ml Lactated Ringers Solution to infuse in 60 min
   Label: Cefoxitin Sodium 2 Gm
   Directions: Reconstitute with 20 ml sterile water for injection to yield 2 Gm/21 ml.
   Drop factor: 60 gtt/ml
   What should the flow rate be?

7. **Order:** Ampicillin Sodium 250 mg IVPB in 100 ml D5W to infuse in 60 min
   Label: Ampicillin Sodium 1 Gm
   Directions: Reconstitute with 3.5 ml sterile water for injection to yield 1 Gm/4 ml.
   Drop Factor: 10 gtt/ml
   a. How many ml of the reconstituted solutions should be added to the IV solution?

b. What should the flow rate be?

8. **Order:** Coly-Mycin M 100 mg in 500 ml D5W to infuse at 5 mg/hr
   Label: Coly-Mycin M (colistimethate sodium) 150 mg
   Directions: Reconstitute with 2 ml sterile water for injection to yield
   75 mg/ml and add to IV solution.
   Drop factor: 60 gtt/ml
   a. How many ml of reconstituted solution should be added to the
   IV solution?

b. What should the flow rate be?

9. **Order:** Mithracin 1534 mcg in 1000 ml D5W to infuse in 6 hr
   Label: Mithracin (plicamycin) 2.5 mg
   Directions: Reconstitute with 4.9 ml of sterile water for injection to
   yield 0.5 mg/ml and add to IV solution.
   Drop Factor: 60 gtt/ml
   a. How many ml of reconstituted Mithracin should be added to the
   ordered IV solution?

b. What should the flow rate be?

10. **Order:** Penicillin G Potassium 5 million units in 100 ml D5W IV to
 infuse over 1 hr
 Label: Penicillin G Potassium 20,000,000 U dry powder
 Directions: Reconstitute with 31.6 ml sterile water for injection to
 yield concentration of 500,000 U/ml.
 Drop Factor: 15 gtt/ml
 a. How many ml of the reconstituted Penicillin G should be added
 to the 100 ml D5W?

 b. What should the flow rate be?

(*Note:* See Appendix C for answer key.)

Adding Drugs to IVs and Calculating the Drug Infusion Rate

The physician may order the IV medication to be infused at the rate of
a specified concentration (amount) of drug per unit of time. We call this
the drug infusion rate.

 The drug infusion rate can be calculated in terms of either:
 a. *volume of solution* per unit of time (e.g., ml/hr or ml/min)
 OR
 b. *concentration of drug* per unit of time (e.g., mg, mcg, U/hr or min).

Example: A drug infusion rate of 2.5 U/hr means that:

 a. the IV flow rate (volume/unit of time) that will infuse 2.5 U of the
 drug per hour must be determined
 OR
 b. the concentration of drug contained in a specified amount of solution
 per hour must be determined.

 Because these are usually potent drugs that require the most accurate
method of infusion, they are administered using a microdrip infusion set
and volumetric infusion pump. Because the pump ml/hr rate corresponds
to the microdrip/min rate, the IV flow rate can be calculated in ml/hr
and the corresponding gtt/min setting selected (see Table 10-1). This will
automatically infuse the correct amount per hour or per minute.

Examples:

a. **Order:** Heparin 20,000 U in 500 ml Sodium Chloride 0.9% IV to infuse at 1200 U/hr. Use an infusion pump.

How many ml/hr should be administered?

Starting Factor   Answer Label
1 hr   ml

Equivalents: 1200 U = 1 hr   20,000 U = 500 ml

Conversion Equation: $1 \text{ hr} \times \dfrac{1200 \text{ U}}{1 \text{ hr}} \times \dfrac{500 \text{ ml}}{20,000 \text{ U}} = 30 \text{ ml}$

Flow Rate: 30 ml/hr

Set the infusion pump at the gtt/min setting that corresponds to 30 ml/hr.

b. **Order:** Heparin 20,000 U in 500 ml Sodium Chloride 0.9% IV to infuse at 30 ml/hr.

How many Units will be infused per hour?

Starting Factor   Answer Label
1 hr   U

Equivalents: 30 ml = 1 hr   20,000 U = 500 ml

Conversion Equation: $1 \text{ hr} \times \dfrac{30 \text{ ml}}{1 \text{ hr}} \times \dfrac{20,000 \text{ U}}{500 \text{ ml}} = 1200 \text{ U}$

c. **Order:** Aminophylline 280 mg in 350 ml D5W into central venous catheter. Infuse 250 ml in 75 min and the remainder at 20 ml/hr. Use an infusion pump.

Label: See Figure 10-20

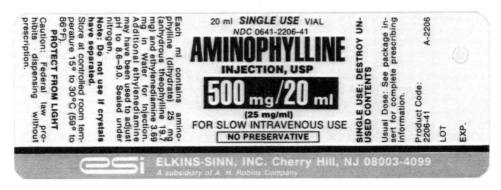

Figure 10-20 (*Courtesy Elkins-Sinn, Inc., A Subsidiary of A. H. Robins Company*)

1. How many ml of medication should be added to the IV bottle?
   Equivalents: 500 mg = 20 ml

   Conversion Equation: $280 \, \cancel{mg} \times \dfrac{20 \, ml}{500 \, \cancel{mg}} = 11.2 \, ml$

   Answer: Add Aminophylline 11.2 ml to 350 ml D5W.

2. How many mg would the patient receive per minute at the infusion rate of 250 ml/75 min?
   Equivalents: 250 ml = 75 min   350 ml = 280 mg

   Conversion Equation: $1 \, \cancel{min} \times \dfrac{250 \, \cancel{ml}}{75 \, \cancel{min}} \times \dfrac{280 \, mg}{350 \, \cancel{ml}} = 2.7 \, mg$

3. Determine the ml/hr to which the infusion pump should be set to infuse the first 250 ml of IV solution at the ordered rate.
   Equivalents: 60 min = 1 hr   250 ml = 75 min

   Conversion Equation: $1 \, \cancel{hr} \times \dfrac{60 \, \cancel{min}}{1 \, \cancel{hr}} \times \dfrac{250 \, ml}{75 \, \cancel{min}} = 200 \, ml$

   Answer: Regulate the infusion pump to deliver 200 ml/hr.

4. How long will it take to infuse the remaining solution at the ordered rate?
   Equivalent: 20 ml = 1 hr

   Conversion Equation: $100 \, \cancel{ml} \times \dfrac{1 \, hr}{20 \, \cancel{ml}} = 5 \, hr$

Practice: Calculation of The Volume of Solution or Concentration of Drug

1. **Order:** Pitocin 25 U in 1000 ml Sodium Chloride 0.9% IV to infuse at a drug infusion rate of 2.5 U/hr
   Label: Pitocin (oxytocin) 10 U/ml
   a. How many ml of Pitocin must be added to the IV bottle?

b. How many ml/hr should be administered?

2. **Order:** Regular Insulin 100 U in 500 ml Sodium Chloride 0.9% to infuse at 5 U/hr via IV pump
   How many ml/hr should be administered?

3. **Order:** Morphine Sulfate 100 mg in 250 ml D5W to infuse at 3.2 mg/hr via IV pump
   How many ml/hr should be administered?

4. **Order:** Heparin 20,000 U in 1000 ml Sodium Chloride 0.9% to infuse at 1000 U/hr via IV pump
   How many ml/hr should be administered?

5. **Order:** Minocin (minocycline) 100 mg in 500 ml D5W to infuse at 20 mg/hr via IV pump
   How many ml/hr should be administered?

6. **Order:** Coly-Mycin-M 150 mg in 100 ml D5W to infuse in 60 minutes
(via IV mini-bottle/saline lock)
Label: Coly-Mycin-M (colestimethate sodium) 150 mg
Directions: Reconstitute with 2 ml sterile water for injection to yield
75 mg/ml and add to ordered amount of IV solution.
How many ml/hr should be administered?

7. **Order:** Cefizox 1 Gm in 50 ml Ringers Solution IV to infuse in 30
min via IV pump
Label: Cefizox (ceftizoxime sodium) 1 Gm
Directions: Reconstitute with 10 ml sterile water for injection to yield
1 Gm/10.7 ml.
How many ml/hr should be administered via the IV pump?

8. **Order:** Pyopen 3 Gm in 100 ml D5W into central venous catheter
to infuse in 90 min (use an infusion pump)
Label: Pyopen (carbenicillin disodium) 5 Gm
Directions: Reconstitute with 7 ml sterile water for injection to yield
500 mg/ml.
a. How many ml of reconstituted solution should be added to the
IV solution?

b. How many ml/hr should be administered via the IV pump?

9. **Order:** Cleocin 300 mg IV (Buretrol) in 50 ml D5W to infuse at dose
rate of 30 mg/min (use an infusion pump)
Label: Cleocin (clindamycin) 300 mg/2 ml
Directions: Dilute in 50 ml of D5W and administer via volume control set.
a. Determine the ml/hr to which the infusion pump should be set.

b. At this rate, how many minutes will it take to infuse the ordered
50 ml?

10. **Order:** Aminophylline 500 mg in 500 ml D5W in 10 hr via IV pump
How many mg will infuse in 1 hr?

11. **Order:** Lidocaine 2 Gm in 500 ml D5W to infuse at 60 ml/hr via
IV pump
How many mg will infuse in 1 min?

12. **Order:** Isuprel (isoproterenol HCl) 2 mg in 500 ml D5W to infuse
at 45 ml/hr via IV pump
How many mcg will infuse in 1 min?

13. **Order:** KCl 10 mEq in 1000 ml D5½NS to infuse at 125 ml/hr via
IV pump
How many mEq will infuse in 1 hr?

14. **Order:** Dopamine 400 mg in 250 ml D5W to infuse at 60 ml/hr via
IV pump
How many mg will infuse in 1 hr?

15. **Order:** Aminophylline 250 mg in 250 ml D5W into central venous
catheter. Infuse 200 ml in 45 minutes and the remainder at
17 ml/hr. Use an IV pump.
Label: Aminophylline 250 mg/10 ml
a. How many ml of medication should be added to the IV bottle?

b. Determine the ml/hr to which the IV pump should be set to infuse
the first 200 ml of solution at the ordered rate.

c. How long will it take to infuse the remaining solution at the ordered rate?

16. **Order:** Magnesium Sulfate 20 Gm in 1000 ml D5W IV via pump. Infuse 600 ml in 90 min and the remainder (400 ml) at 50 ml/hr

    Label: Magnesium Sulfate 5 Gm/10 ml

    a. How many ml should be added to the IV?

    b. How many Gm would the patient receive per minute at the infusion rate of 600 ml/90 min?

    c. Determine the ml/hr to which the IV pump should be set to infuse the first 600 ml of solution at the ordered rate.

    d. How long will it take to infuse the remaining solution at the ordered rate?

17. **Order:** Ritadrine Hydrochloride 150 mg in 500 ml Ringers IV (via IV pump) to infuse at 0.1 mg/min and increase by 0.05 mg/min every 10 min until uterine contractions cease

    Label: Ritadrine HCl 50 mg/5 ml

    a. How many ml of the medication should be added to the IV bottle?

b. What is the concentration of the resulting solution per ml (i.e., mg of Ritadrine/ml)?

c. How many ml/hr should be administered to infuse the initial dose of 0.1 mg/min?

d. Ten minutes later, the flow rate should be increased to how many ml/hr to infuse the ordered dose (0.1 mg + 0.05 mg = 0.15 mg)?

e. Ten minutes later, the flow rate should be increased to how many ml/hr to infuse the ordered dose (0.15 mg + 0.05 mg = 0.2 mg)?

(*Note:* See Appendix C for answer key.)

Calculating IV Dosage and Flow Rate Based on Body Weight

IV medications may be ordered according to a *specified amount* (e.g., mcg/kg of body weight) to be administered within a *specified unit* of time (e.g., per minute). The medication is added to a *specified volume and type* of IV solution. The total desired dose per minute must first be determined and then the infusion rate calculated that will administer the correct ml/hr or gtt/min. As a rule, a microdrip infusion set (60 gtt/ml) is used, along with an IV pump or controller.

Examples:
  a. **Order:** Infuse Nipride (nitroprusside sodium) 50 mg in 500 ml D5W
        at 3 mcg/kg/min
  Weight: 215 lb
  Drop Factor: 60 gtt/ml
  1. How many mcg/min must be administered?

$$215 \,\cancel{lb} \times \frac{1 \,\cancel{kg}}{2.2 \,\cancel{lb}} \times \frac{3 \,\text{mcg/min}}{1 \,\cancel{kg}} = 293.2 \,\text{mcg/min}$$

  2. How many ml/hr will provide the required dose?

$$1 \,\cancel{hr} \times \frac{60 \,\cancel{min}}{1 \,\cancel{hr}} \times \frac{293.2 \,\cancel{mcg}}{1 \,\cancel{min}} \times \frac{1 \,\cancel{mg}}{1000 \,\cancel{mcg}} \times \frac{500 \,\text{ml}}{50 \,\cancel{mg}} = 175.9$$
$$= 176 \,\text{ml/hr}$$

  3. How many gtt/min will provide the required dose?

$$1 \,\cancel{min} \times \frac{293.2 \,\cancel{mcg}}{1 \,\cancel{min}} \times \frac{1 \,\cancel{mg}}{1000 \,\cancel{mcg}} \times \frac{500 \,\cancel{ml}}{50 \,\cancel{mg}} \times \frac{60 \,\text{gtt}}{1 \,\cancel{ml}} = 175.9$$
$$= 176 \,\text{gtt/min}$$

OR

$$215 \,\cancel{lb} \times \frac{1 \,\cancel{kg}}{2.2 \,\cancel{lb}} \times \frac{3 \,\cancel{mcg}}{1 \,\cancel{kg}} \times \frac{1 \,\cancel{mg}}{1000 \,\cancel{mcg}} \times \frac{500 \,\cancel{ml}}{50 \,\cancel{mg}} \times \frac{60 \,\text{gtt}}{1 \,\cancel{ml}} = 175.9$$
$$= 176 \,\text{gtt/min}$$

  4. How many mcg/gtt will be administered?

$$1 \,\cancel{gtt} \times \frac{1 \,\cancel{min}}{176 \,\cancel{gtt}} \times \frac{293.2 \,\text{mcg}}{1 \,\cancel{min}} = 1.7 \,\text{mcg/gtt}$$

Note: When calculating gtt/min, the step of calculating mcg/min can
be omitted.
  b. **Order:** Infuse Heparin 10,000 U in 250 ml D5W at 0.4 U/kg/min
  Weight: 59 kg
  Drop Factor: 60 gtt/ml
  1. How many U/min must be administered?

$$59 \,\cancel{kg} \times \frac{0.4 \,\text{U/min}}{1 \,\cancel{kg}} = 23.6 \,\text{U/min}$$

  2. How many ml/hr will provide the required dose?

$$1 \,\cancel{hr} \times \frac{60 \,\cancel{min}}{1 \,\cancel{hr}} \times \frac{23.6 \,\cancel{U}}{1 \,\cancel{min}} \times \frac{250 \,\text{ml}}{10,000 \,\cancel{U}} = 35 \,\text{ml/hr}$$

3. How many gtt/min will provide the required dose?

$$1\,\text{min} \times \frac{23.6\,\text{U}}{1\,\text{min}} \times \frac{250\,\text{ml}}{10,000\,\text{U}} \times \frac{60\,\text{gtt}}{1\,\text{ml}} = 35\,\text{gtt/min}$$

OR

$$59\,\text{kg} \times \frac{0.4\,\text{U}}{1\,\text{kg}} \times \frac{250\,\text{ml}}{10,000\,\text{U}} \times \frac{60\,\text{gtt}}{1\,\text{ml}} = 35\,\text{gtt/min}$$

4. How many U/gtt will be administered?

$$1\,\text{gtt} \times \frac{1\,\text{min}}{35\,\text{gtt}} \times \frac{23.6\,\text{U}}{1\,\text{min}} = 0.7\,\text{U/gtt}$$

Practice: IV Flow Rate and Dosages Based on Body Weight

1. **Order:** Infuse Amrinone 250 mg in 500 ml D5W at 5 mcg/kg/min
   Weight: 202 lb
   Drop Factor: 60 gtt/ml
   a. How many mcg/min must be administered?

   b. How many ml/hr will provide the required dose?

   c. How many gtt/min will provide the required dose?

   d. How many mcg/gtt will be administered?

2. **Order:** Infuse Dobutamine 250 mg in 250 ml D5W at 7 mcg/kg/min
   Weight: 73.6 kg
   Drop Factor: 60 gtt/ml
   a. How many mcg/min must be administered?

   b. How many ml/hr will provide the required dose?

   c. How many gtt/min will provide the required dose?

   d. How many mcg/gtt will be administered?

3. **Order:** Infuse Nitroprusside 50 mg in 250 ml D5W at 1.5 mcg/kg/min
   Weight: 198 lb
   Drop Factor: 60 gtt/ml

    a. How many mcg/min must be administered?

    b. How many ml/hr will provide the required dose?

    c. How many gtt/min will provide the required dose?

    d. How many mcg/gtt will be administered?

4. **Order:** Intropin (dopamine HCl) 800 mg in 250 ml D5W at 8 mcg/
       kg/min
  Weight: 72.8 kg
  Drop Factor: 60 gtt/ml
  a. How many mcg/min must be administered?

b. How many ml/hr will provide the required dose?

c. How many gtt/min will provide the required dose?

d. How many mcg/gtt will be administered?

5. **Order:** Infuse Dobutamine 250 mg in 150 ml D5W at 5 mcg/kg/min
   Weight: 83.2 kg
   Drop Factor: 60 gtt/ml
   a. How many mcg/min must be administered?

b. How many ml/hr will provide the required dose?

c. How many gtt/min will provide the required dose?

d. How many mcg/gtt will be administered?

(*Note:* See Appendix C for answer key.)

Tritrated Infusions

Some very potent drugs are administered according to the patient's physiologic responses to the medication. That is, the dose is increased or decreased until the desired effect has been achieved. This effect may be: raising or lowering the blood pressure, controlling arrhythmias or seizures, relieving chest pain, or treating other often life-threatening situations.

The technique of adjusting dose/flow rate to obtain a precise desired effect is called *titration*. Examples of drugs administered by titration include: dopamine, nitroprusside, nitroglycerine, lidocaine, oxytocin, and magnesium sulfate.

Titrated drugs are given IV, either continuous or intermittent, depending on the volume and/or frequency of administration and equipment available. Small volume infusions may be administered via syringe or saline lock, and large volume infusions via an IV line, usually with a controlled volume set and always using an infusion pump.

Titration calculations are based on: solution concentration, infusion rate, and concentration of drug (i.e., mg/min, mcg/min, units/min, and mcg/kg/min). In addition, calculation of the *titration (or concentration) factor* (i.e., the concentration of drug per drop) (e.g., mg/gtt, μg/gtt, etc.) determines the exact amount of drug infusing any time a flow rate adjustment is made. The gtt/min may be increased or decreased depending on the patient's response to the current flow rate. The titration factor (drug/gtt) is used to determine the drug concentration (drug/min) provided by the adjusted flow rate.

Titrated drug orders may be written as a range of dosage between which the therapeutic dosage for an individual should fall (e.g., 5–10 mcg/kg/min). Therefore, the calculations involve determining the upper and lower therapeutic doses and titrating the dose within these limits. These calculations should be compared with the safe dose range recommended by the manufacturer.

Because titrated infusions require frequent dosage adjustments, it follows that the infusion pump settings must be readjusted simultaneously. Because of the minute changes in drug concentrations, it is essential that microdrip tubing be used. Therefore, the drop factor for calculating adjusted flow rates always will be 60 gtt/ml.

Several steps are necessary for calculating titrated infusions. Each step can be performed by using the label-factor method, thus eliminating the need to memorize a confusing array of formulas. Each of the following steps has been presented in the preceding section; they are now arranged in the correct sequence for titration.

Steps in calculating titrated infusions:

1. Determine the concentration (drug/ml) of the solution to be administered.
2. Determine the amount of drug/min that will administer the ordered range of titration.
3. Determine how many ml/hr or gtt/min will administer the ordered range of titration.
4. Determine the titration (concentration) factor in drug/gtt.
5. If necessary, increase or decrease the gtt/min and determine the adjusted dosage (drug/min) the patient is receiving.

Continue titrating until the desired effect is achieved.

Example:

Order: Infuse Nipride (nitroprusside) 50 mg in 250 ml D5W. Titrate 3–6 mcg/kg/min to maintain the systolic blood pressure at 150 mm Hg
Weight: 135 lb
   a. What is the concentration of the solution in mcg/ml?
      Equivalents: 50 mg = 250 ml   1 mg = 1000 mcg

$$\text{Conversion Equation: } 1 \, \cancel{ml} \times \frac{50 \, \cancel{mg}}{250 \, \cancel{ml}} \times \frac{1000 \, mcg}{1 \, \cancel{mg}} = 200 \, mcg/ml$$

   b. How many mcg/min will administer the ordered range of titration?
      Lower (3 mcg/kg/min):
      Equivalents: 1 kg = 2.2 lb   1 kg = 3 mcg/min

$$\text{Conversion Equation: } 135 \, \cancel{lb} \times \frac{1 \, \cancel{kg}}{2.2 \, \cancel{lb}} \times \frac{3 \, mcg/min}{1 \, \cancel{kg}} = 184 \, mcg/min$$

Upper (6 mcg/kg/min):
Equivalents: 1 kg = 2.2 lb   1 kg = 6 mcg/min

Conversion Equation: $135 \, \cancel{lb} \times \dfrac{1 \, \cancel{kg}}{2.2 \, \cancel{lb}} \times \dfrac{6 \, mcg/min}{1 \, \cancel{kg}} = 368 \, mcg/min$

The range of dosage for this patient is 184–368 mcg/min.

  c. How many ml/hr or gtt/min will administer the ordered range of titration?

Lower:
Equivalents: 1 hr = 60 min   1 min = 184 mcg   200 mcg = 1 ml

Conversion Equation: $1 \, \cancel{hr} \times \dfrac{60 \, \cancel{min}}{1 \, \cancel{hr}} \times \dfrac{184 \, \cancel{mcg}}{1 \, \cancel{min}} \times \dfrac{1 \, ml}{200 \, \cancel{mcg}}$
$$= 55 \, ml/hr \text{ or } 55 \, gtt/min$$

Upper:
Equivalents: 1 hr = 60 min   1 min = 368 mcg/min   200 mcg = 1 ml

Conversion Equation: $1 \, \cancel{hr} \times \dfrac{60 \, \cancel{min}}{1 \, \cancel{hr}} \times \dfrac{368 \, \cancel{mcg}}{1 \, \cancel{min}} \times \dfrac{1 \, ml}{200 \, \cancel{mcg}}$
$$= 110 \, ml/hr \text{ or } 110 \, gtt/min$$

The range of ml/hr and gtt/min for this IV is 55–110 ml/hr or 55–110 gtt/min.

  d. What is the titration (concentration) factor in mcg/gtt?
Equivalents: 55 gtt = 1 min   184 mcg = 1 min

Conversion Equation: $1 \, \cancel{gtt} \times \dfrac{1 \, \cancel{min}}{55 \, \cancel{gtt}} \times \dfrac{184 \, mcg}{1 \, \cancel{min}} = 3.3 \, mcg/gtt$

  e. The present systolic blood pressure reading is 170 mm Hg. Increase the gtt/min by 5 gtt. How many mcg/min will the patient now be receiving?
Equivalents: 1 min = 60 gtt   1 gtt = 3.3 mcg

Conversion Equation: $1 \, \cancel{min} \times \dfrac{60 \, \cancel{gtt}}{1 \, \cancel{min}} \times \dfrac{3.3 \, mcg}{1 \, \cancel{gtt}} = 198 \, mcg/min$

  f. After 1 hr, the systolic blood pressure reading is 120 mm Hg. Decrease the gtt/min by 6 gtt. How many mcg/min will the patient now be receiving?
Equivalents: 1 min = 54 gtt   1 gtt = 3.3 mcg

Conversion Equation: $1 \, \cancel{min} \times \dfrac{54 \, \cancel{gtt}}{1 \, \cancel{min}} \times \dfrac{3.3 \, mcg}{1 \, \cancel{gtt}} = 178.2 \, mcg/min$

Practice: Titration Infusions

1. **Order:** Infuse Esmolol HCl 5 Gm in 500 ml D5W. Titrate 50–100 mcg/kg/min to maintain the systolic blood pressure at 120 mm Hg.

   Weight: 140 lb

   a. What is the concentration of the solution in mcg/ml?

   b. How many mcg/min will administer the ordered range of titration?
   Lower (50 mcg/kg/min):

   Upper (100 mcg/kg/min):

   c. How many ml/hr or gtt/min will administer the ordered range of titration?
   Lower:

   Upper:

    d. What is the titration (concentration) factor in mcg/gtt?

    e. The present systolic blood pressure reading is 160 mm Hg. Increase the gtt/min by 5 gtt. How many mcg/min will the patient now be receiving?

2. **Order:** Infuse Dopamine 400 mg in 500 ml D5W. Titrate 5–10 mcg/kg/min to maintain the systolic blood pressure greater than 100 mm Hg.
Weight: 175 lb
    a. What is the concentration of the solution in mcg/ml?

    b. How many mcg/min will administer the ordered range of titration?
    Lower (5 mcg/kg/min):

    Upper (10 mcg/kg/min):

c. How many ml/hr or gtt/min will administer the ordered range of titration?
Lower:

Upper:

d. What is the titration (concentration) factor in mcg/gtt?

e. The present systolic blood pressure reading is 68 mm Hg. Increase the gtt/min by 10 gtt. How many mcg/min will the patient now be receiving?

3. **Order:** Infuse Amrinone lactate 250 mg in 50 ml NS. Titrate 5–10 mcg/kg/min to maintain the diastolic blood pressure below 90 mm Hg.
Weight: 70 kg
a. What is the concentration of the solution in mcg/ml?

b. How many mcg/min will administer the ordered range of titration?
Lower (5 mcg/kg/min):

Upper (10 mcg/kg/min):

c. How many ml/hr or gtt/min will administer the ordered range of titration?
Lower:

Upper:

d. What is the titration (concentration) factor in mcg/gtt?

e. The present diastolic blood pressure reading is 100 mm Hg. Increase the gtt/min by 5 gtt. How many mcg/min will the patient now be receiving?

4. **Order:** Infuse Nitropress (nitroprusside sodium) 50 mg in 500 ml
     D5W. Titrate 1.5–3 mcg/kg/min to maintain the systolic blood
     pressure at 100 mm Hg.
   Weight: 200 lb
   a. What is the concentration of the solution in mcg/ml?

   b. How many mcg/min will administer the ordered range of titration?
      Lower (1.5 mcg/kg/min):

      Upper (3 mcg/kg/min):

   c. How many ml/hr or gtt/min will administer the ordered range of
      titration?
      Lower:

      Upper:

d. What is the titration (concentration) factor in mcg/gtt?

e. The present systolic blood pressure reading is 90 mm Hg. Decrease the gtt/min by 5 gtt. How many mcg/min will the patient now be receiving?

5. **Order:** Infuse Dopamine Hydrochloride 200 mg in 500 ml D5W. Titrate 2–5 mcg/kg/min to maintain the systolic blood pressure at a minimum of 100 mm Hg.
   Weight: 165 lb
   a. What is the concentration of the solution in mcg/ml?

b. How many mcg/min will administer the ordered range of titration?
   Lower (2 mcg/kg/min):

Upper (5 mcg/kg/min):

c. How many ml/hr or gtt/min will administer the ordered range of titration?
Lower:

Upper:

d. What is the titration (concentration) factor in mcg/gtt?

e. The present systolic blood pressure reading is 80 mm Hg. Increase the gtt/min by 5 gtt. How many mcg/min will the patient now be receiving?

(*Note:* See Appendix C for answer key.)

Drugs Administered by IV Bolus

When a small amount of medication is injected directly into a vein, it is called an IV bolus or IV push. A venipuncture can be performed in any accessible vein and the medication injected by means of a syringe. If an IV is already in place, the medication can be injected through a Y-port or the flashball at the end of the infusion tubing. An IV bolus also can be given through the saline lock. Some infusion pumps are designed to deliver an IV bolus at a controlled rate.

Because drugs given by IV bolus will have an immediate effect, the rate of injection becomes extremely important. Administering IV injections too quickly can result in adverse side effects and/or speed shock. Many drugs are ordered to be injected over a period of 1–30 minutes. On the other hand, some drugs must be given rapidly, even within a period of seconds, because an immediate effect is desired or necessary. It is, therefore, essential to determine the correct IV injection rate and to time this accurately using a clock or wristwatch with a second hand. The need for precision in this regard cannot be overemphasized.

Example:

Order: Chloromycetin 300 mg IV bolus via saline lock
Label: Chloromycetin (chloramphenicol) 1 Gm
Directions: Reconstitute with 10 ml sterile water for injection to yield 100 mg/ml. Safe injection rate is 1 Gm/min.

  a. How many ml of Chloromycetin should be administered?
     Equivalents: 1 Gm = 10 ml   1000 mg = 1 Gm

$$\text{Conversion Equation: } 300 \, \text{mg} \times \frac{1 \, \text{Gm}}{1000 \, \text{mg}} \times \frac{10 \, \text{ml}}{1 \, \text{Gm}} = 3 \, \text{ml}$$

  b. How long should it take to administer this IV bolus?
     Equivalents: 1 Gm = 10 ml   1000 mg = 1 Gm

$$\text{Conversion Equation: } 3 \, \text{ml} \times \frac{1 \, \text{Gm}}{10 \, \text{ml}} \times \frac{1 \, \text{min}}{1 \, \text{Gm}} = 0.3 \, \text{min} = 18 \, \text{seconds}$$

OR

$$300 \, \text{mg} \times \frac{1 \, \text{Gm}}{1000 \, \text{mg}} \times \frac{1 \, \text{min}}{1 \, \text{Gm}} = 0.3 \, \text{min} = 18 \, \text{seconds}$$

Practice: IV Bolus

1. **Order:** Emete-Con 20 mg IV bolus via 3-way stopcock of infusion tubing
    Label: Emete-Con 50 mg
    Directions: Reconstitute with 2.2 ml of sterile water for injection to yield a concentration of 25 mg/ml. Safe injection rate is 25 mg/30 sec. (The apparent discrepancy here between amount of added diluent and amount of resulting solution is explained by the *hydrophilic* property of Emete-Con, i.e., possessing the ability to absorb moisture.)
  a. How many ml should be injected?

b. How long should it take to administer this IV bolus?

2. **Order:** Aminophylline 240 mg IV bolus via saline lock
   Label: Aminophylline 25 mg/ml
   Directions: Do not exceed rate of 25 mg/min for IV bolus.
   a. How many ml of Aminophylline should be administered?

   b. What is the least number of minutes required to administer this IV bolus of Aminophylline into the saline lock?

3. **Order:** Digoxin 0.5 mg IV bolus via primary infusion line
   Label: Digoxin 0.25 mg/ml
   Directions: Do not exceed rate of 0.25 mg/min for IV bolus.
   a. How many ml of Digoxin should be administered?

   b. What is the least number of minutes it should take to administer this IV bolus of Digoxin?

4. **Order:** Demerol 30 mg IV bolus via Y-tube/primary line
   Label: Demerol (meperidine) 50 mg/ml
   Directions: Do not exceed rate of 25 mg/min for IV bolus.
   a. What is the total amount of solution to be injected?

   b. How long should it take to administer this IV bolus?

5. **Order:** Lasix 35 mg IV bolus via saline lock
   Label: Lasix (furosemide) 10 mg/ml
   Directions: Administer undiluted. Maximum injection rate = 20
              mg/min.
   a. What is the total amount of solution to be injected?

   b. How long should it take to administer this IV bolus?

6. **Order:** Bretylium 5 mg/kg IV bolus
   Label: Bretylium 500 mg/ml
   Directions: Do not exceed injection rate of 25 mg/min.
   a. How many mg should be administered via bolus (patient weighs
      135 lb)?

b. How many ml would the bolus contain?

c. How long should it take to administer this bolus?

7. **Order:** Lidocaine 1 mg/kg IV bolus. Follow by Lidocaine drip 1000 mg/250 ml of D5W and run at 2 mg/min.
   Label: Bolus-Lidocaine (1%) 10 mg/ml
   Label: IV-Lidocaine (20%) 200 mg/ml
   Directions: Do not exceed injection rate of 35 mg/min.
   a. How many mg of Lidocaine (1%) would be administered via bolus (patient weighs 170 lb)?

   b. How many ml would the bolus contain?

   c. How long should it take to administer this bolus?

d. How many ml of Lidocaine (20%) should be added to the IV?

e. How many ml/hr should be administered IV?

(*Note:* See Appendix C for answer key.)

Parenteral Nutrition

When nutritional needs cannot be met by enteral intake, supplementary or total nutrition can be provided via parenteral routes. Basic nutrients, electrolytes, and vitamins, as well as fluid requirements, can be administered intravenously through a peripheral or central vein. Choice of route depends on tonicity and/or concentration of the solution, as well as anticipated duration of parenteral nutrition administration.

Terms associated with parenteral nutrition include:

TPN: Total Parenteral Nutrition—all nutrients essential for tissue maintenance are provided intravenously.

CPN: refers to IV nutrition via a central vein, usually the superior vena cava. The terms *TPN* and *CPN* often are used interchangeably.

PTPN: Peripheral Total Parenteral Nutrition (or PPN—Peripheral Parenteral Nutrition) refers to IV nutrition via a peripheral vein, usually the radial, basilic, or cephalic vein of the arm.

Hyperalimentation: refers to the provision of nutrients in excess of maintenance needs.

Regardless of the route used for administration, it is important to remember that parenteral nutrition solutions are natural culture mediums for bacterial growth and should not hang in excess of 12 hr.

Nutrition calculations can be used to determine the amounts of nutrients and energy contained in a parenteral nutrition formula (IV solution). Generally, they are concerned with the caloric value, expressed as kilocalories (kcal) of the glucose, amino acid, and/or fat emulsion content of the IV solution.

Equivalents necessary for setting up the conversion equations include:

*1 Gm glucose = 3.4 kcal
1 Gm amino acid (protein) = 4 kcal
1 Gm of 10% fat emulsion = 1.1 kcal
1 Gm of 20% fat emulsion = 2 kcal

In a percentage solution, the symbol % refers to *parts of substance (solid) per 100 parts of solution (liquid)* (i.e., 1 Gm of solid is equivalent to 1 ml of liquid). See Appendix B, Equivalent Units for Solids and Liquids.

Thus: a 5% solution indicates 5 Gm/100 ml
a 2.5% solution indicates 2.5 Gm/100 ml

Note: kcal values for intravenous CHO and fat are different from the kcal values for the same orally ingested nutrients. Protein values are unchanged.

4 kcal/Gm of CHO
4 kcal/Gm of protein
9 kcal/Gm of fat

Examples:

Order: TPN 1000 ml D5W (carbohydrate), 500 ml Liposyn II 10% (fat),
500 ml Aminosyn 3.5% (protein) IV

How many kcal of carbohydrates, fats, and proteins are provided by this IV?

Carbohydrates:
Equivalents: 5 Gm = 100 ml   1 Gm = 3.4 kcal

Conversion Equation: $1000 \, \text{ml} \times \dfrac{5 \, \text{Gm}}{100 \, \text{ml}} \times \dfrac{3.4 \, \text{kcal}}{1 \, \text{Gm}} = 170 \, \text{kcal}$

Fats:
Equivalents: 10 Gm = 100 ml   1 Gm = 1.1 kcal

Conversion Equation: $500 \, \text{ml} \times \dfrac{10 \, \text{Gm}}{100 \, \text{ml}} \times \dfrac{1.1 \, \text{kcal}}{1 \, \text{Gm}} = 55 \, \text{kcal}$

Protein:
Equivalents: 3.5 Gm = 100 ml   1 Gm = 4 kcal

Conversion Equation: $500 \, \text{ml} \times \dfrac{3.5 \, \text{Gm}}{100 \, \text{ml}} \times \dfrac{4 \, \text{kcal}}{1 \, \text{Gm}} = 70 \, \text{kcal}$

Practice: Nutrition Calculations

1. **Order:** TPN 1500 ml D5W IV
   How many kcal of carbohydrate are provided?

2. **Order:** TPN 1000 ml Aminosyn 3.5% IV
   How many kcal of protein are provided?

3. **Order:** CPN 1000 ml Liposyn II 10% IV
   How many kcal of fat are provided?

4. **Order:** TPN 500 ml 2.5% Dextrose in Water IV
   How many kcal of carbohydrate are provided?

5. **Order:** PTPN 1500 ml Aminosyn PF 7% IV
   How many kcal of protein are provided?

6. **Order:** TPN 2500 ml D10W IV
   How many kcal of carbohydrate are provided?

7. **Order:** CPN 1500 ml Intralipid 20% IV
   How many kcal of fat are provided?

8. **Order:** TPN 3000 ml 20% Dextrose in Water IV
   How many kcal of carbohydrate are provided?

9. **Order:** TPN 1000 ml Aminosyn II 5% and 500 ml 25% Dextrose in
   Water IV
   a. How many kcal of protein are provided?

   b. How many kcal of carbohydrates are provided?

10. **Order:** TPN 1000 ml Aminosyn II 4.25% and 1000 ml D10W IV

   a. How many kcal of protein are provided?

   b. How many kcal of carbohydrate are provided?

   (*Note:* See Appendix C for answer key.)

Assessment and Adjustment

One of the major responsibilities of the nurse who is caring for patients with intravenous infusions is observation and assessment. The flow rate is assessed by counting the drops per minute (gtt/min) and determining what adjustments need to be made in the event the rate has changed. A checklist, such as the example in Figure 10-21, may be useful in performing the IV assessment.

A variety of factors can affect the flow rate including positional changes that may alter the angle of the needle or catheter, a clot that partially obstructs the infusion flow, improper height of the container, tubing dangling below insertion site, dislodgement of needle or clamp, and infiltration or irritation at the insertion site.

Regardless of the infusion system used (e.g., gravity (plain IV), controller, or pump), nursing assessment is of prime importance, because early observation and correction of undesirable factors are essential to maintain the infusion at the designated rate and to prevent adverse occurrences. Even if the IV is attached to an automatic infusion pump or controller, frequent observation is necessary to be sure the system is working properly and the desired flow rate is being maintained.

IV ASSESSMENT

Pt. Initials _____   Room # _____

Name of IV fluid being infused _____

_____

#ml left in bag/bottle _____

Drip rate: _____ cc/hr or _____ gtt/min

Without disturbing dressing, what is condition of IV site? _____

_____

What time do you anticipate IV bag/bottle will need to be changed? _____

What IV solution will be hung next? _____

Figure 10-21   IV assessment

Although the previous section dealt with use of the label factor method to calculate the initial flow rate, most nurses will be much more frequently involved with maintaining IV infusions than starting them. This involves periodic observation of the amount of fluid remaining to be infused and re-calculation of the flow rate to determine if adjustments need to be made to complete the IV within the ordered time period. The label factor method lends itself equally well to determining the need for adjustment of the flow rate when any of the previously mentioned factors have caused it to speed up or slow down.

Example:

■ **Starting IV:**
   Order: 1000 ml of Sodium Chloride 0.9% to infuse over a period of 8 hr.
   Drop Factor: 15 gtt/ml
   Question: What should the flow rate be when the IV is started?

   Answer: $1 \, \text{min} \times \dfrac{1 \, \text{hr}}{60 \, \text{min}} \times \dfrac{1000 \, \text{ml}}{8 \, \text{hr}} \times \dfrac{15 \, \text{gtt}}{1 \, \text{ml}} = 31 \, \text{gtt}$

■ **Assessing the IV:**

After the IV has been running 5 hr, there are still 450 ml left to infuse. Does the IV flow rate need to be adjusted to complete the infusion in the ordered time period?

Two factors must be noted in this problem. First, the total amount of solution is now 450 ml; second, the total number of hours remaining is 3.

The conversion equation is written exactly as before, substituting the new values in the conversion factor ml/hr.

$$1 \, \text{min} \times \frac{1 \, \text{hr}}{60 \, \text{min}} \times \frac{450 \, \text{ml}}{3 \, \text{hr}} \times \frac{15 \, \text{gtt}}{1 \, \text{ml}} = 37.5 = 38 \, \text{gtt}$$

■ **Adjusting the IV:**

The IV flow rate must be adjusted to 38 gtt/min.

Remember: Although minor adjustments in flow rate are permissible (usually less than 25% increase over the initial flow rate), larger increases require a physician's order. One exception is in the administration of parenteral nutrition when any flow rate increase could be hazardous. Whenever there is a question, consult the physician.

Practice: Adjusting IVs—(Calculate in gtt/min)

1. **Order:** 2500 ml of D5W IV to infuse over a period of 12 hr
   Drop Factor: 10 gtt/ml
   a. What should the flow rate be when the IV is started?

   b. After the IV has been running 8 hours, there are still 800 ml left to infuse. To what should the flow rate be adjusted to have the IV completed on schedule?

2. **Order:** 1000 ml Lactated Ringers IV in 6 hr
   Drop Factor: 15 gtt/ml
   a. What should the initial flow rate be?

   b. After 4 hr, 350 ml remain. To what should the flow rate be adjusted to have the IV completed on schedule?

3. **Order:** 3000 ml D5W IV in 24 hr
   Drop Factor: 20 gtt/ml
   a. What should the initial flow rate be?

   b. After 18 hr, 600 ml remain. What should the adjusted flow rate be?

4. **Order:** 1500 ml D2.5W IV in 12 hr
   Drop Factor: 10 gtt/ml
   a. What should the initial flow rate be?

b. After 7 hr, 800 ml remain. What should the adjusted flow rate be?

5. **Order:** 500 ml Sodium Chloride 0.9% IV in 8 hr
   Drop Factor: 60 gtt/ml
   a. What should the initial flow rate be?

b. After 5 hr, 150 ml remain. What should the adjusted flow rate be?

6. **Order:** 750 ml Ringers IV in 4 hr
   Drop Factor: 10 gtt/ml
   a. What should the initial flow rate be?

b. After 2 ½ hr, 300 ml remain. What should the adjusted flow rate be?

7. **Order:** 2000 ml D5W IV in 18 hr
   Drop Factor: 15 gtt/ml
   a. What should the initial flow rate be?

   b. After 11 hr, 900 ml remain. What should the adjusted flow rate be?

8. **Order:** 250 ml Isolyte M IV in 5 hr
   Drop Factor: 60 gtt/ml
   a. What should the initial flow rate be?

   b. After 2 hr, 120 ml remain. What should the adjusted flow rate be?

9. **Order:** 1250 ml D2.5NS IV in 9 hr
   Drop Factor: 15 gtt/ml
   a. What should the initial flow rate be?

b. After 3 hr, 750 ml remain. What should the adjusted flow rate be?

10. **Order:** 125 ml Sodium Chloride 0.9% in 2 hr IV
     Drop Factor: 60 gtt/ml
     a. What should the initial flow rate be?

b. After 1 ½ hr, 30 ml remain. What should the adjusted flow rate be?

(*Note:* See Appendix C for answer key.)

Administration of Intravenous Medications and Solutions

•••

Objectives

Upon completion of this unit of study you should be able to:
- *Identify safe and suitable sites for intravenous injections and infusions.*
- *Identify nursing responsibilities in relation to administering, assessing, and monitoring intravenous injections and infusions.*
- *Follow infection-control guidelines with respect to safe handling or manipulation of IV equipment.*
- *Identify performance criteria related to IV medications and solutions.*

Intravenous Administration

A variety of methods can be used when medications or fluids are given intravenously. The traditional method has been the gravity infusion system. This method, commonly referred to as "an IV," is called a continuous infusion and is employed for the purpose of providing or replacing fluids directly into the blood, rather than via the gastrointestinal route. Medications can be added to this continuous IV for slow administration or can be infused directly into the intravenous line for more rapid administration. The latter is called intermittent infusion and may be administered via IV piggy back, a volume control set, a saline lock, or a central venous catheter; medications also can be injected directly into a vein by means of an IV bolus (push).

Although nurses increasingly are assuming responsibility for starting IVs and administering IV medications, these activities require specialized knowledge and are regulated by nurse practice acts and agency policy. Nurses should be aware of their professional and legal responsibilities with respect to intravenous administration.

Infusion Sites

Any easily accessible vein may be chosen for venipuncture. Most commonly used are the hand and lower arm, the antecubital fossa, and the upper arm, Figure 11-1. Less desirable are veins in the legs and feet, because of the greater risk of thrombophlebitis and embolism. A central venous line may be used for infusion directly through a major vein such as the subclavian. In infants, a scalp vein often is used.

When veins are inaccessible or very difficult to reach, a venisection may be required. In this procedure, called a cut-down, the skin is incised to expose a vein for insertion of the IV needle.

Nursing Responsibilities Relative to Intravenous Administration

In addition to the principles for administration of medications listed in Units 7 and 9, specific nursing responsibilities in relation to intravenous injections and infusions include the following:

■ Setting up for an intravenous infusion: obtaining correct solution, infusion set, and needle; attaching and priming tubing; adding medica-

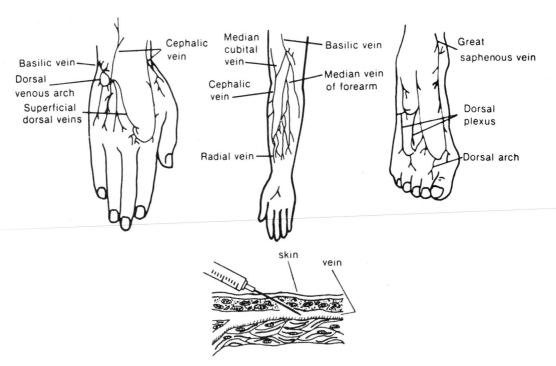

Figure 11-1 Continuous gravity intravenous infusion

tion if ordered; and labeling container appropriately (e.g., patient's name, solution, rate, date, and time).

■ Positioning patient comfortably, explaining procedure, preparing venipuncture site: shaving, immobilizing, etc.

■ Performing venipuncture, initiating intravenous infusion, adjusting flow rate, and terminating infusion upon completion.

■ Monitoring the intravenous infusion by maintaining flow rate as ordered. The rate of flow should be checked by counting the number of drops per minute at least every 30 min or more often if necessary, even if an IV pump or controller is in use. If this is done, the ordered flow rate can be maintained with very minor adjustments being required. It is important to keep in mind the risks associated with too slow or too rapid administration of intravenous solutions. (*Note:* The flow rate may be checked by counting the drop rate for 15 sec and multiplying by 4.)

■ Checking patency of the system, placement of needle or intracatheter and condition of site; attaching additional containers of fluid as ordered; noting and recording amount of fluid administered.

■ Administering medication through the IV.

■ Changing IV dressing and/or IV tubing as necessary or according to hospital policy.

■ Providing physical care for the patient including assistance with meals, ambulation, comfort, and hygiene.

■ Observing for complications associated with intravenous administration:
  1. Fluid overload resulting from too rapid administration of intravenous solutions.
     Signs: —rapid breathing
            —shortness of breath
            —dilation of neck veins
            —increase in blood pressure
            —decreased fluid output in relation to fluid intake
  2. Speed shock resulting from too rapid administration of intravenous medication, especially bolus injection.
     Signs: —headache
            —flushed face
            —irregular pulse
            —decrease in blood pressure (shock)
     (*Note:* The nurse should use caution in increasing the IV flow rate even if it is running behind schedule. Speeding up the IV in an attempt to catch up and complete in the specified time could cause fluid overload or speed shock. If major adjustments in flow rate are deemed necessary, a physician's order should be obtained.)

3. Infiltration (leakage) of IV solution into subcutaneous tissue surrounding venipuncture site due to displacement of needle or intracatheter.
   Signs: —sluggish flow rate
   —absence of blood backflow
   —localized swelling, pallor, pain
   —area cool to touch

4. Thrombophlebitis (injury or irritation to a vein) resulting in clot formation at end of needle or intracatheter.
   Signs: —sluggish flow rate
   —redness, pain, heat at IV site and/or along affected vein

5. Allergic reaction to IV fluid or additive.
   Signs: —rash
   —itching
   —shortness of breath

6. Infection at venipuncture site related to improper care of IV site (i.e., dressing changes, etc.).
   Signs: —discharge
   —inflammation

7. Systemic infection related to contamination of equipment or solutions.
   Signs: —elevated TPR
   —chills, malaise

8. Air embolism resulting from air in tubing due to loose connections or containers running dry. (*Note:* More common when an infusion pump is being used.)
   Signs: —cyanosis
   —hypotension
   —weak, rapid pulse
   —loss of consciousness

9. Catheter embolism resulting from improper insertion, accidental breakage, or dislodgement.
   Signs: same as air embolism, plus discomfort in involved vein

Precautions in Handling IV Equipment

Because the administration of IV fluids and medications involves the risk of coming into contact with blood and/or body fluids, it is essential that:

■ sterile technique be maintained in performing venipuncture, changing site dressings, and manipulating any equipment that subjects the patient to the risk of infection.

■ personnel observe blood and body fluid precautions as recommended by the Centers for Disease Control. This includes wearing gloves when

flushing lumens, terminating IVs, or performing any procedure that subjects personnel to a risk of infection through contact with blood or body fluids.
■ all needles used in administration of intravenous therapy be discarded into puncture-resistant containers.

Recording

Intravenous medications and solutions are recorded in a variety of locations depending on policies of the agency. These may include the Medex, a special intravenous form, nurses notes, and/or the intake/output record. The initial notation should include information relative to time, type, site, and flow rate. Subsequent notations document ongoing assessment, observations, flow rate, additives, patient's response, adverse effects, and time of termination.

Performance Criteria: Setting Up an IV

The learner is referred to a nursing text or skills manual for detailed instruction on performance of venipuncture and administration of continuous intravenous infusion. The following checklists may be helpful as a guide for intravenous administration.

	S	U	Comments
1. Washes hands			
2. Gathers equipment a) Bottle or bag of prescribed IV solution			
b) Proper tubing (vented or non-vented)			
c) IV pole			
3. Examines the container a) Correct solution			
b) Correct amount			
c) Expiration date			
d) Glass bottle, intact			
e) Plastic bag (absence of dimples or puncture marks)			
f) Solution, clear			

Continued on next page

Performance Criteria: Setting Up an IV *(Cont.)*

	S	U	Comments
4. Examines the tubing a) Spike cover, intact and secure			
5. Slides flow clamp along tubing until it is directly under drip chamber and closes the clamp			
6. Spikes the container a) Bottle with rubber stopper (uses vented tubing). Removes metal cap, swabs stopper with alcohol; places bottle on stable surface, steadies by holding stopper between finger and thumb; removes plastic cover from spike and pushes spike firmly into rubber stopper, avoiding contamination; hangs on IV pole			
b) Bottle with indwelling vent and a latex diaphragm (uses non-vented tubing). Removes protective metal cap and diaphragm; notes release of vacuum; inserts spike in proper opening; hangs on IV pole			
c) Plastic bag (uses non-vented tubing). Hangs on IV pole before spiking; steadies port with one hand and removes protective cap by pulling smoothly to the right; inserts spike into port with one quick motion			
7. Gently squeezes drip chamber until half full (or full, depending on equipment instructions)			
8. Primes the tubing a) Holds end over sink, wastebasket, etc.			

Continued on next page

Performance Criteria: Setting Up an IV (Cont.)

	S	U	Comments
b) Removes protective cap, without contaminating inside (does not discard cap)			
c) Unclamps tubing and lets fluid run through until it fills the tubing and all air bubbles have been expelled. Maintains sterility of end of tubing			
d) If small bubbles appear at top of tubing or in drip chamber, lightly taps area until bubbles rise into chamber			
e) Clamps off tubing and replaces protective cap			
9. Loops tubing over IV pole until ready to perform venipuncture			
10. Labels container and tubing with date, time of insertion and any medication added			

S—Satisfactory   U—Unsatisfactory   Evaluator _____

Performance Criteria: Starting IV (with an Over-the-Needle Type Catheter)

	S	U	Comments
1. Washes hands			
2. Obtains equipment and sets up IV			
3. Prepares patient for procedure			
4. Selects vein; shaves site if necessary			
5. Applies tourniquet			
6. Puts on gloves			
7. Preps insertion site with antiseptic			

Continued on next page

Performance Criteria: Starting IV (with an Over-the-Needle Type Catheter) (Cont.)

	S	U	Comments
8. Removes protective shield from catheter set			
9. Grasps patient's arm so that the thumb below the insertion site increases skin tension and stabilizes the vein			
10. Places needle at 30° angle with bevel up, about 1 cm distal to venipuncture site			
11. Punctures the skin so that the needle approaches the vein from the side			
12. Advances the needle into the vein at a slight angle to the vein, with slow, steady pressure			
13. Aligns the needle with the vein and follows the vein until about an eighth of an inch of the plastic catheter is within the lumen			
14. After blood flows into the body of the catheter releases thumb pressure on patient's arm, holds the metal needle firmly in place with one hand and advances the plastic catheter smoothly into the vein			
15. Continues to advance the catheter until the catheter hub is approximately one-fourth inch from the puncture site			
16. Loosens the tourniquet, holds the catheter steady, withdraws and discards metal needle into puncture-resistant container as soon as possible			
17. Removes cap from the IV tubing and joins the catheter and tubing adapters firmly together			

Continued on next page

Performance Criteria: Starting IV (with an Over-the-Needle Type Catheter) (Cont.)

	S	U	Comments
18. Opens the clamp on the IV tubing to a fast rate to check for free-flow, then partially closes clamp			
19. Tapes the catheter hub to the patient's arm			
20. Applies dressing in such a manner that dressing can be changed without disturbing the catheter			
21. Forms a loose loop in the tubing and tapes to patient's arm			
22. Adjusts the IV flow to the prescribed rate			
23. Indicates the size of the needle and date on the tape			
24. Secures an armboard in such a manner that circulation and comfort are not impaired			

S—Satisfactory   U—Unsatisfactory   Evaluator _____

Performance Criteria: Assessment, Adjustment, and Termination of IV

	S	U	Comments
1. Assesses by observing a) patency of tubing			
b) rate of flow			
c) amount remaining			
d) injection site			
e) patient's reaction			
2. Adjusts flow rate to correct number of drops/minute			

Continued on next page

Performance Criteria: Assessment, Adjustment, and Termination of IV (Cont.)

	S	U	Comments
3. Terminates when indicated, applying principles of asepsis, safety, and comfort a) puts on gloves			
b) clamps off			
c) loosens tape			
d) places sterile gauze pad over site			
e) withdraws needle, immediately applies pressure and elevates limb			
f) discards needle into puncture-resistant container			
g) maintains pressure as necessary			
h) applies band-aid securely			

S—Satisfactory   U—Unsatisfactory   Evaluator _____

Pediatric Dosage

....

Objectives

Upon completion of this unit of study you should be able to:
- *Identify special considerations related to safety and comfort when administering medications to infants and children.*
- *Identify adaptations and special considerations related to administration of oral and parenteral medications to infants and children when giving intramuscular injections and intravenous infusions.*
- *Apply the label factor method to clinical calculations of pediatric dosage based on body weight and body surface area.*

There are several methods for calculating pediatric medication dosage based on various combinations of age, height, weight, body surface area, and adult dose. Because children of the same age can vary widely in size and weight, most of the usual methods are not applicable in all cases. Furthermore, rules or formulas do not take into consideration the physical condition of the child and the variety of responses and/or susceptibilities to the effects of drugs possible in individual children. Because of the serious consequences that may result from overdosage or underdosage, accuracy of calculating and precision of administering medications to infants and children is of prime importance.

General Considerations in Administering Oral and Parenteral Medications to Children

■ Be sure positive identification has been made by comparison of name tag with medication administration guide or other means. Do not rely on child's response to spoken name.

■ Corroborate calculated dosages by double-checking with another nurse and/or referring to a drug information source. This is particularly important when administering insulin, heparin, or digoxin.

■ Exercise particular caution in maintaining security of drugs, medication cart, needles, syringes, etc., making sure they are not accessible to children.

- Be sure child is awake and alert before administering oral medications. Never administer oral medications to a crying or resisting child or an injection to a sleeping child.
- Make explanations according to child's developmental level of understanding regarding reasons for medication, route of administration, expected sensations, taste, etc. Allow child to express feelings; be accepting of negative reactions.
- Maintain a firm, but friendly manner. Give praise and comfort following administration.
- Restrain child gently, but firmly. Obtain assistance as necessary, particularly for injections.
- Children up to 3 years of age are unable to swallow pills, and even older children may have much difficulty. Crush and dissolve pills and tablets (exclusive of enteric coated) as necessary. Administer liquids via cup, spoon, dropper, or syringe. For infants, medications can be placed in an empty nipple, from which the infant can suck.

Administration of Parenteral Medications to Infants and Children

Intramuscular Injections

The site of choice for intramuscular injections in infants and children under the age of 3 is the lateral aspect of the thigh, the vastus lateralis muscle. The reason for this is that in children under the age of 3 years, the gluteal muscle is very small and poorly developed, and injection in this area is dangerously close to the sciatic nerve.

The ventrogluteal site is acceptable in children over 3 years who have been walking for 1 year or more, and is a good site because it is free of major nerves and blood vessels. Figure 12-1 illustrates the method for locating this site. The thumb is placed on the anterior superior iliac spine and the index finger is abducted posteriorly. The injection site is located between the thumb and index finger. The dorsogluteal site should be avoided until the child is over age 4.

In older children, over age 5, the deltoid muscle is an acceptable site as long as the number and volume of injections is limited.

Special consideration must be given to safety aspects of administering injections. Needles with a smaller diameter and shorter length should be used. For most infants and small children, a 25 gauge, 1″ needle is preferable unless solution is too viscous. Children must be restrained to avoid injury. A mummy restraint is suitable for infants; older children can be gently, but firmly restrained by the person giving the injection or by another individual, if necessary. Make explanations brief, give injections quickly but safely, and allow the child to cry or express feelings. It is especially important for the nurse or parent to pick up, soothe, and comfort infants and young children following an injection.

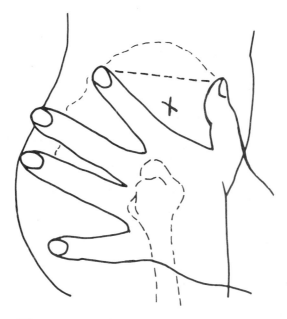

Figure 12-1   Ventrogluteal site in child

Intravenous Infusions

Because infants have such small arm and hand veins, scalp veins (temporal area) or the superior longitudinal sinus often are chosen as intravenous sites. In young children, the external jugular vein is an acceptable alternative site. When a scalp vein is used, the area must be shaved. It is important to avoid cuts during shaving, because of the danger of infection. A scalp vein needle is securely taped in place and covered with a gauze dressing. Additional protection such as a small plastic or paper cup is necessary to prevent dislodgement.

In young children, acceptable intravenous sites are the veins on the dorsal surface of the hand or flexor surface of the wrist; also the leg and foot veins. The antecubital site is used least often, because of the difficulty of preventing dislodgement.

Infants and young children must be restrained adequately during insertion of the needle and the duration of the infusion. Mummy and/or elbow restraints and sandbags are effective methods. Armboards or other immobilizing devices may be used for older children.

Intravenous infusions must be checked as often as every 15–30 minutes. Because of the greater risk of fluid overload, an automatic rate-flow infusion pump always should be used to regulate and maintain the rate of flow. A pediatric infusion set featuring volume control is an additional safety measure to prevent IV fluid overload by allowing only 50–100 ml of solution into the fluid chamber at one time. The minidrip feature of the volume control infusion set allows for easier regulation of the flow rate and more precise intravenous administration. A syringe-pump (mini-infuser) is useful in administering small amounts of intravenous fluids at a controlled rate. It is essential to maintain an accurate record of fluid intake and output on children receiving IV infusions.

Pediatric Dosage Based on Body Weight—Oral Medications

Examples:

a. **Order:** Digoxin Elixir Pediatric 15 mcg/kg of body weight/dose po
   Label: Digoxin 0.05 mg/ml
   Weight: 60 lb
   How many ml should the child receive per dose?
   Starting Factor   Answer Label
         60 lb   ml
   Equivalents: 1 kg = 2.2 lb   15 mcg = 1 kg
                 1000 mcg (μg) = 1 mg   0.05 mg = 1 ml

Conversion Equation:

$$60 \text{ lb} \times \frac{1 \text{ kg}}{2.2 \text{ lb}} \times \frac{15 \text{ mcg}}{1 \text{ kg}} \times \frac{1 \text{ mg}}{1000 \text{ mcg}} \times \frac{1 \text{ ml}}{0.05 \text{ mg}} = 8.2 \text{ ml}$$

b. **Order:** Coly-Mycin S 5 mg/kg of body weight/day po to be given in
           3 divided doses
   Label: Coly-Mycin S (Colestimethate sodium) 25 mg/5 ml
   Weight: 4.5 kg
   How many drops should be administered per dose?
   Equivalents: 25 mg = 5 ml, 5 mg = 1 kg, 15 gtt = 1 ml, 3 doses =
              4.5 kg

Conversion Equation:

$$4.5 \text{ kg} \times \frac{5 \text{ mg}}{1 \text{ kg}} \times \frac{5 \text{ ml}}{25 \text{ mg}} \times \frac{15 \text{ gtt}}{1 \text{ ml}} = \frac{67.5 \text{ gtt}}{3 \text{ doses}} = 22.5 = 23 \text{ gtt}$$

Because it is important to administer the exact amount ordered, the computation should be carried out to two decimal places and rounded to the nearest tenth. To obtain a more precise measurement than is possible with a medicine cup, the medication should be measured using a syringe. It then may be administered directly from the syringe.

Practice: Calculating Pediatric Dosage Based on Body Weight—Oral Medications

1. **Order:** Lanoxin Elixir 30 µg/kg/dose po
   Label: Figure 12-2. What is the generic name? _____
   Weight: 28 lb
   How many ml should the child receive?

2. **Order:** Amoxicillin Suspension 20 mg/kg in three divided doses/day po
   Label: Figure 12-3
   Weight: 44 lb
   How many ml should be administered per dose?

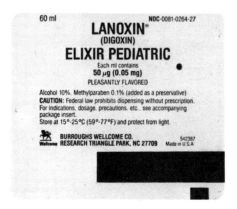

Figure 12-2 *(Courtesy Burroughs Wellcome Co.)*

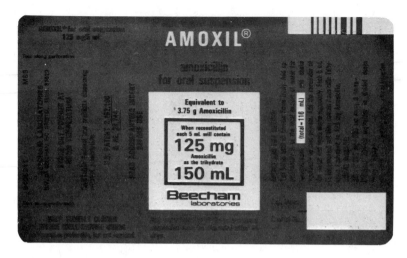

Figure 12-3   (*Courtesy Beecham Laboratories*)

3. **Order:** Gantrisin Pediatric Suspension 150 mg/kg po in four divided
      doses/day
   Label: Gantrisin Pediatric Suspension (sulfasoxizole) 0.5 Gm/tsp
   Weight: 40 lb
   How many ml should be administered per dose?

4. **Order:** Somophylin Oral Liquid 2.5 mg/lb/dose po
   Label: Somophylin (aminophylline) Oral Liquid 90 mg/tsp
   Weight: 18 kg
   How many ml should the child receive per dose?

5. **Order:** Omnipen Oral Suspension 50 mg/kg/day in four divided
      doses po
   Label: Omnipen (ampicillin) Oral Suspension 125 mg/5 ml
   Weight: 33 lb
   How many ml should be administered per dose?

6. **Order:** Velosef Expectorant 25 mg/kg in two divided doses po
   Label: Velosef (cephradine) Expectorant 250 mg/5 ml
   Weight: 44 lb
   How many ml should be administered per dose?

7. **Order:** Tetracycline Syrup 25 mg/kg/day in four divided doses po
   Label: Tetracycline Syrup 125 mg/5 ml
   Weight: 37 kg
   How many ml should be administered per dose?

8. **Order:** Amcill Pediatric Drops 50 mg/kg/day in four divided doses po
   Label: Amcill (ampicillin) Pediatric Drops 125 mg/5 ml
   Weight: 42 lb
   How many ml should be administered per dose?

9. **Order:** Antiminth Oral Suspension 5 mg/lb single dose po
   Label: Antiminth (pyrantil pamoate) Oral Suspension 50 mg/ml
   Weight: 45 lb
   How many ml should be administered per dose?

10. **Order:** Cleocin Pediatric 8 mg/kg/day in four divided doses po
    Label: Cleocin (clindamycin) Pediatric 75 mg/5 ml
    Weight: 84 lb
    How many ml should be administered per dose?

11. **Order:** Elixophyllin Elixir 0.3 ml/lb/dose po
    Label: Elixophyllin (theophylline) Elixir 80 mg/15 ml
    Weight: 44 lb
    How many ml should be administered per dose?

12. **Order:** Furadantin Oral Suspension 5 mg/kg in four divided doses po
    Label: Furadantin (nitrofurantoin) Oral Suspension 25 mg/5 ml
    Weight: 15 lb
    How many ml should be administered per dose?

13. **Order:** Pentids 56 mg/kg/day in six divided doses po
    Label: Pentids (penicillin G potassium) Oral Suspension 125
    mg/5 ml
    Weight: 38 lb
    How many ml should be administered per dose?

14. **Order:** Penbritin Pediatric Drops Oral Suspension 5 mg/lb/dose po
    Label: Penbritin (ampicillin) Pediatric Drops Oral Suspension 100
    mg/ml
    Weight: 12 lb
    How many ml should be administered per dose?

15. **Order:** Pfizerpen G 25,000 U/kg/day in three divided doses po
    Label: Pfizerpen G (penicillin G potassium) 400,000 U/5 ml
    Weight: 20 kg
    How many ml should be administered per dose?

16. **Order:** Principen 250 Oral Suspension 50 mg/kg/day in four divided
    doses po
    Label: Principen 250 (ampicillin) Oral Suspension 250 mg/ml
    Weight: 20 kg
    How many ml should be administered per dose?

(*Note:* See Appendix C for answer key.)

Calculating Pediatric Dosage—Injections

Example:

Order: Bicillin LA 50,000 U/kg/day IM in four divided doses
Label: Bicillin LA (penicillin G Benzathine) 300,000 U/ml
Weight: 50 lb
How many ml will be administered per dose?
Equivalents: 1 kg = 2.2 lb, Bicillin LA 300,000 U = 1 ml, 50,000 U = 1 kg

Conversion Equation:

$$50 \; \cancel{lb} \times \frac{1 \; \cancel{kg}}{2.2 \; \cancel{lb}} \times \frac{50,000 \; \cancel{U}}{1 \; \cancel{kg}} \times \frac{1 \; ml}{300,000 \; \cancel{U}} = \frac{3.78 \; ml}{4 \; doses} = 0.95 \; ml = 1 \; ml$$

(*Note:* When the resulting dosage is less than 1 ml, the answer may be carried to three decimal places and rounded to the nearest hundredth, and the medication may be measured and administered in a tuberculin syringe. If the dosage is 1 ml or more, carry the answer to two decimal places and round to the nearest tenth.)

**Practice: Calculating Pediatric Dosage—Injections
(see note above)**

1. **Order:** Kanamycin Sulfate Injection 15 mg/kg/in two divided doses/
    day IM
    Label: Figure 12-4. What is the trade name? _____
    Weight: 5 kg
    How many ml should the child receive per dose?

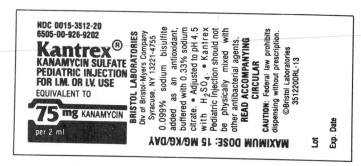

Figure 12-4 (*Courtesy Bristol-Myers U.S. Pharmaceutical Group, Evansville, IN 47721*)

2. **Order:** Lasix 3 mg/kg IM
   Label: Figure 12-5. What is the generic name? _____
   Weight: 25 lb
   How many ml should the child receive?

3. **Order:** Keflin 100 mg/kg/day in four divided doses IM
   Label: Keflin (cephalothin) 500 mg/2.2 ml
   Weight: 15 lb
   How many ml should the child receive per dose?

4. **Order:** Streptomycin 30 mg/kg/day in two divided doses IM
   Label: Streptomycin 1 Gm/2 ml
   Weight: 20 lb
   How many ml should the child receive per dose?

Lasix®
(furosemide)
Injection IM/IV
For Single Use Only
10 mL Vial
10 mL = 100 mg(10 mg/mL)

Caution: Federal law prohibits dispensing without prescription.

Manufactured for:
HOECHST-ROUSSEL
Pharmaceuticals Inc.
Somerville, N.J. 08876
REG. TM HOECHST AG
65710285

Store at controlled room temperature (59°-86°F).
Do not use if solution is discolored.

LOT 0570028
EXP. OCT. 89

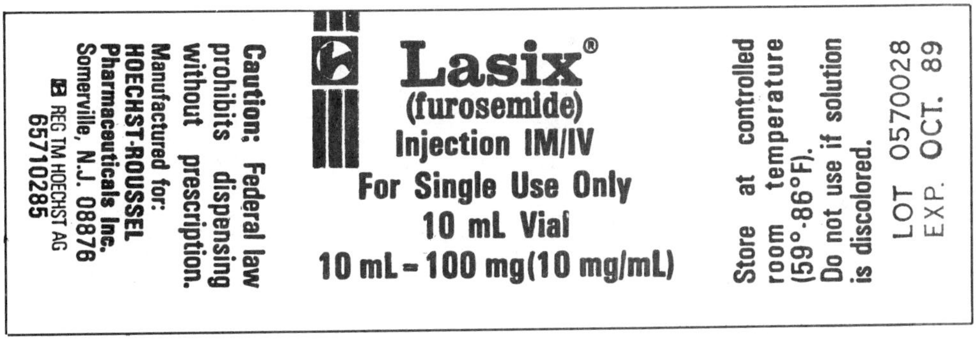

Figure 12-5   (*Courtesy Hoechst-Roussel Pharmaceuticals Inc.*)

5. **Order:** Polycillin-N 150 mg/kg/day in six divided doses IM
   Label: Polycillin-N (ampicillin) 250 mg/ml
   Weight: 55 lb
   How many ml should the child receive per dose?

6. **Order:** Apresoline 1.7 mg/kg/day in four divided doses IM
   Label: Apresoline (hydralazine HCl) 20 mg/ml
   Weight: 12 lb
   How many ml should the child receive per dose?

7. **Order:** Humatrope 0.06 mg/kg/day IM
   Label: Humatrope (somatropin) 5 mg/4 ml
   Weight: 12.2 kg
   How many ml should the child receive per dose?

8. **Order:** Penicillin G Potassium 35,000 U/kg/day in four divided
   doses IM
   Label: Penicillin G Potassium 250,000 U/ml
   Weight: 72 lb
   How many ml should the child receive per dose?

9. **Order:** Rocephin 50 mg/kg/day in two divided doses IM
   Label: Rocephin (cetriaxone) 250 mg/ml
   Weight: 22.7 kg
   How many ml should the child receive per dose?

10. **Order:** Digoxin 0.002 mg/kg/day in two divided doses IM
    Label: Digoxin 0.5 mg/2 ml
    Weight: 25 lb
    How many ml should the child receive per dose?

(*Note:* See Appendix C for answer key.)

Calculating Pediatric Dosage—IVs

Example:

Order: Dopamine 5 mcg/kg/min IV. Dilute 100 mg Dopamine in 100
 ml D5½NS
Label: Figure 12-6
Weight: 10 lb

| EXP. | LOT | NDC 0641-**0112-25** 25 x **5 mL** *Single Use* Vials **DOPAMINE** HCl INJECTION, USP **200 mg/5 mL** (40 mg/mL) FOR IV INFUSION ONLY | **POTENT DRUG: MUST DILUTE BEFORE USING** Each mL contains dopamine hydrochloride 40 mg (equivalent to 32.3 mg dopamine base) and sodium bisulfite 10 mg in Water for Injection. pH 2.5-5.0. Sealed under nitrogen. USUAL DOSE: See package insert. Do not use if solution is discolored. Store at 15° - 30° C (59° - 86° F). Caution: Federal law prohibits dispensing without prescription.   B-50112c |

ELKINS-SINN, INC. Cherry Hill, NJ 08003-4099
A subsidiary of A. H. Robins Company

Figure 12-6   (*Courtesy Elkins-Sinn, Inc., A Subsidiary of A. H. Robins Company*)

a. How many ml of Dopamine should be added to the 100 ml D5½NS to obtain the ordered dilution?

$$100 \text{ mg} \times \frac{5 \text{ ml}}{200 \text{ mg}} = 2.5 \text{ ml}$$

b. How many mcg of Dopamine should the child receive per min?

$$10 \text{ lb} \times \frac{1 \text{ kg}}{2.2 \text{ lb}} \times \frac{5 \text{ mcg/min}}{1 \text{ kg}} = 22.7 \text{ mcg/min}$$

c. How many mcg of Dopamine should the child receive per hr?

$$1 \text{ hr} \times \frac{60 \text{ min}}{1 \text{ hr}} \times \frac{22.7 \text{ mcg}}{1 \text{ min}} = 1362 \text{ mcg}$$

d. What should the flow rate be in ml/hr to infuse the calculated dose?

$$1 \text{ hr} \times \frac{1362 \text{ mcg}}{1 \text{ hr}} \times \frac{1 \text{ mg}}{1000 \text{ mcg}} \times \frac{100 \text{ ml}}{100 \text{ mg}} = 1 \text{ ml}$$

OR

$$1 \text{ hr} \times \frac{60 \text{ min}}{1 \text{ hr}} \times \frac{22.7 \text{ mcg}}{1 \text{ min}} \times \frac{1 \text{ mg}}{1000 \text{ mcg}} \times \frac{100 \text{ ml}}{100 \text{ mg}} = 1 \text{ ml}$$

e. The infusion pump would be set at an automatic flow rate of 1 ml/hr. Assuming that a microdrip infusion set is being used, what would be the gtt/hr?   60

Practice: Calculating Pediatric Dosage—IVs

1. **Order:** Lidocaine 30 mcg/kg/min IV. Dilute 300 mg Lidocaine in 250 ml D5W

   Label: Lidocaine 1 Gm/25 ml

   Weight: 32.6 kg

   a. How many ml of Lidocaine should be added to the 250 ml D5W to obtain the ordered dilution?

b. How many mcg of Lidocaine should the child receive per min?

c. How many mg of Lidocaine should the child receive per hr?

d. What should the flow rate be in ml/hr to infuse the calculated dose?

e. At the calculated rate, how many hours should it take for the total IV to infuse?

2. **Order:** Nitropress 2 mcg/kg/min IV. Dilute 30 mg in 250 ml D5½NS
   Label: Nitropress (nitroprusside sodium) 50 mg/2 ml
   Weight: 18.5 kg
   a. How many ml of Nitropress should be added to the 250 mg D5½NS to obtain the ordered dilution?

b. How many mcg of Nitropress should the child receive per min?

c. How many mg of Nitropress should the child receive per hr?

d. What should the flow rate be in ml/hr to infuse the calculated dose?

3. **Order:** Aminophylline 0.3 mg/kg in 30 ml D5W IV to infuse over 20 min
   Label: Figure 12-7
   Weight: 45 lb
   a. How many mg should the child receive as a total dose?

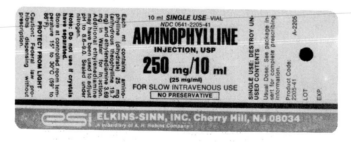

Figure 12-7 (*Courtesy Elkins-Sinn, Inc., A Subsidiary of A. H. Robin. Company*)

b. How many ml of Aminophylline should be added to the 30 ml D5W?

4. **Order:** Verapamil Hydrochloride 0.2 mg/kg via IV bolus
   Label: Verapamil Hydrochloride 5 mg/2 ml
   Weight: 10 lb
   Directions: Administer over a 2 min period.
   How much solution should be administered per dose?

5. **Order:** Isoptin 0.3 mg/kg via IV bolus
   Label: Isoptin (verapamil HCl) 5 mg/2 ml
   Weight: 60 lb
   Directions: Administer over a 2 min period.
   How much solution should be administered per dose?

6. **Order:** Monistat IV 20 mg/kg. Administer IV in three divided doses
   Label: Monistat IV (miconazole) 200 mg/20 ml
   Weight: 40 lb
   Directions: Dilute in 200 ml Sodium Chloride 0.9%. Infuse each dose
            in 60 minutes.
   Drop Factor: 60 gtt/ml
   a. How many ml of Monistat IV will contain the ordered dose?

b. What should the flow rate be?

7. **Order:** Tagamet 5 mg/kg IV in 100 ml D5W. Infuse in 20 min
   Label: Tagamet (cimetidine) 300 mg/2 ml
   Weight: 50 lb
   Drop Factor: 60 gtt/ml
   a. How much Tagamet should be added to the 100 ml D5W?

b. What should the flow rate be?

8. **Order:** Cosmegen 0.015 mg/kg IV in 50 ml D5W. Administer in 15 min
   Label: Cosmegen (dactinomycin) 0.5 mg/ml
   Weight: 64 lb
   Drop Factor: 60 gtt/ml
   a. How much Cosmegen should be added to the 50 ml D5W?

b. What should the flow rate be?

(*Note:* See Appendix C for answer key.)

Calculation of Pediatric Dosage Based on Body Surface Area

Pediatric dosage can be calculated on the basis of the body surface area of the child, which can be determined by the use of a nomogram, Figure 12-8. This method can be used for children up to 12 years of age. The

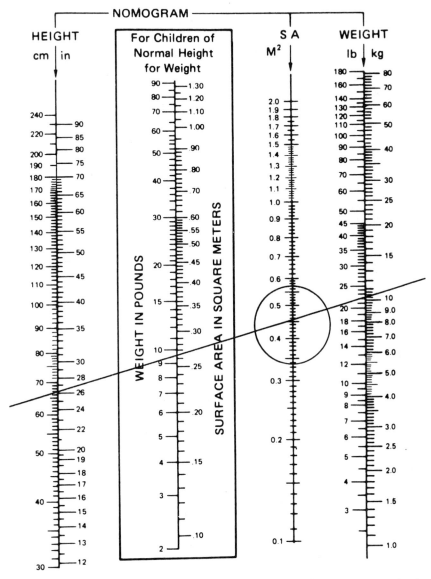

Figure 12-8 (*Modified from* Nelson's Textbook Pediatrics (12th Ed.) *by R. Behrman and V. Vaughan. Copyright by W. B. Saunders Company, Philadelphia, PA*)

child's weight and height are located on the chart; a straight line drawn between them intersects the body-surface column (SA) at the number indicating the child's body surface area (BSA). The surface area measurement is expressed in square meters (M^2). This figure is then plugged into a modified label factor equation, Figure 12-9, to calculate pediatric dosage using BSA estimates.

The child's body surface area in M^2 is located on the nomogram (Figure 12-8) in the following manner: Child's height: 26 in
Child's weight: 22 lb

Place a ruler at the level of the child's weight (22 lb) in the right-hand column and line the edge up with the child's height (26 in) in the left-hand column. Read the surface-area (SA) measurement at the point where the ruler intersects the SA column. The body surface area for this child is 0.45 M^2.

The enclosed (center) column on the nomogram can be used as an estimate of body surface of children of average height and/or build using weight alone.

Practice: Use the Nomogram to Determine the Child's Body Surface Area

1. Child's height: 149 cm
   Child's weight: 36 kg
   Body surface area: _____
2. Child's height: 46 in
   Child's weight: 44 lb
   Body surface area: _____
3. Child's height: 138 cm
   Child's weight: 32 kg
   Body surface area: _____
4. Child's height: 29 in
   Child's weight: 22 lb
   Body surface area: _____
5. Child's height: 82 cm
   Child's weight: 12 kg
   Body surface area: _____

(*Note:* See Appendix C for answer key.)

$$\text{Child's BSA (M}^2) \times \frac{\text{Adult Dose}}{1.7 \text{ M}^2} = \underline{\hspace{2cm}} \text{ (Child's Dose)}$$

Figure 12-9   BSA label factor conversion equation

Application of Label Factor Method Using BSA Estimates

From the BSA label factor conversion equation, Figure 12-9, it can be seen that the equivalent relationship between *average adult body surface area* (1.7 M^2) and *adult dose* becomes a conversion factor or bridge whereby the *child's BSA* (M^2) and the *child's dose* also become an equivalent relationship.

Example: Find the child's dose of Amoxicillin
        Adult dose: Amoxicillin 250 mg
        Child's height: 104 cm
        Child's weight: 9.6 kg   From Nomogram: BSA = 0.51 M^2

          Starting Factor   Answer Label
          Child's BSA (M^2)   Child's dose in mg
             0.51 M^2 _____ mg
      Equivalent: 1.7 M^2 = 250 mg

$$\text{Conversion Equation } 0.51 \, \cancel{M^2} \times \frac{250 \text{ mg}}{1.7 \, \cancel{M^2}} = 75 \text{ mg}$$

Practice: Use Nomogram (Figure 12-8) and Label Factor Method to Calculate Pediatric Dosages

(*Note:* Carry to two decimal places and round to nearest tenth.)

1. Child's height: 25 in
   Child's weight: 14 lb
   Adult dose: Meperidine 50 mg
   Find the child's dose.

2. Child's height: 108 cm
   Child's weight: 18 kg
   Adult dose: Mellaril (thioridazine) 10 mg
   Find the child's dose.

3. Child's height: 46 in
   Child's weight: 50 lb
   Adult dose: Xylocaine Hydrochloride 200 mg
   Find the child's dose.

4. Child's height: 54 in
   Child's weight: 70 lb
   Adult dose: Ceftin (cefuroxime) 250 mg
   Find the child's dose.

5. Child's height: 150 cm
   Child's weight: 38 kg
   Adult dose: Augmentin (amoxicillin and potassium clavunate) 250 mg
   Find the child's dose.

(*Note:* See Appendix C for answer key.)

Clinical Calculations

··

Objective

Upon completion of this unit of study you should be able to:
- *Apply the label factor method to solve, with 100% accuracy, any type of clinical calculation involved in the administration of medication.*

The following clinical problems represent the type of calculations that commonly are encountered in the administration of medications. The prescription orders, the label information, and the conversions required are truly representative of clinical practice. Successful completion of these problems would indicate acceptable competence in performing clinical calculations. With the mastery of this systematic, unified method of problem solving, the learner also should have developed a measure of confidence in his/her ability to solve new problems as they may occur in the clinical setting.

Although most of the equivalent relationships should have been memorized by now, it may be helpful to detach the table of equivalents (printed on the back of title page) for use as a reference in completing the following calculations and for future use in the clinical area.

Before beginning this unit, you may wish to review the method (and modifications) for determining the starting factor and answer label.

■ In general, the starting factor is the particular labeled value that is to be converted to an equivalent relationship (quantity of medication).

Example:

Starting Factor	Answer Label
gr, Gm	mg, cap, tsp

■ In calculations based on body weight, the starting factor is the particular quantity of weight that is to be converted to an equivalent relationship (quantity of medication).

Example:

Starting Factor	Answer Label
lb, kg	ml, mg, tab ÷ number of doses

■ In calculations based on body surface area, the starting factor is the particular amount of body surface area that is to be converted to an equivalent relationship (child's dose).

Example:

Starting Factor	Answer Label
BSA (M^2)	mg, ml, gtt

■ In calculations for IV flow rate in gtt/min, the starting factor is the particular amount of time (1 min) that is to be converted to an equivalent relationship (number of drops).

Example:

Starting Factor	Answer Label
min	gtt

■ In calculations for IV flow rate in ml/hr, the starting factor is the particular amount of time (1 hr) that is to be converted to an equivalent relationship (number of ml).

Example:

Starting Factor	Answer Label
hr	ml

■ In calculations for IV infusion time, the starting factor is the particular amount of solution (ml) that is to be converted to an equivalent relationship (amount of time).

Example:

Starting Factor	Answer Label
ml	hr, min, sec

Practice: Solve Using the Label Factor Method

(*Note:* Round in the appropriate manner.)

1. **Order:** Antabuse 250 mg po
   Label: Antabuse (disulfiram) 0.5 Gm/tab (scored)

2. **Order:** Colchicine gr 1/200 po
   Label: Colchicine 0.6 mg/tab (scored)

3. **Order:** Lanoxin 0.125 mg po
   Label: Lanoxin (digoxin) 0.25 mg/tab (scored)

4. **Order:** Dynapen Oral Suspension 125 mg po
   Label: Dynapen (dicloxacillin sodium) Oral Suspension 62.5 mg/
   5 ml

5. **Order:** Prostaphlin 0.5 Gm po
   Label: Prostaphlin (oxacillin sodium) 250 mg caps

6. **Order:** Dramamine 100 mg po
   Label: Dramamine (dimenhydrinate) 50 mg tabs

7. **Order:** Keflex 1 Gm po
   Label: Keflex (cephalexin) 500 mg caps

8. **Order:** Zyloprim 0.3 Gm po
   Label: Zyloprim (allopurinol) 100 mg/tab

9. **Order:** Vibramycin Syrup 125 mg po
   Label: Vibramycin (doxycycline calcium oral suspension) Syrup 50
   mg/tsp
   Give _____ ml

10. **Order:** Codeine Sulfate gr ½ po
    Label: Codeine Sulfate 15 mg tab

11. **Order:** V Cillin K Oral Suspension 125 mg po
    Label: V Cillin K (penicillin V potassium) Oral Suspension 250
    mg/5 ml

12. **Order:** Chloral Hydrate Suspension 0.75 Gm po
    Label: Chloral Hydrate Suspension 0.5 Gm/3i
    Give _____ ml

13. **Order:** Nembutal Elixir 60 mg po
    Label: Nembutal (pentobarbital) Elixir gr 1/3/tsp
    Give _____ ml

14. **Order:** Mysoline Suspension 125 mg po
    Label: Mysoline 0.25 Gm/5 ml (primidone) Suspension 0.25 Gm/5 ml
    Give _____ ml

15. **Order:** Amoxicillin Suspension 350 mg po
    Label: Amoxicillin Suspension 250 mg/5 ml
    Give _____ drops

16. **Order:** Riopan 10 ml po
    Label: Riopan (magaldrate) 400 mg/tsp
    Give _____ mg

17. **Order:** Saluron 0.15 Gm po
    Label: Saluron (hydroflumethiazide) 50 mg/tab

18. **Order:** Klorvess 30 mEq po
    Label: Klorvess (potassium chloride) 20 mEq/15 ml

19. **Order:** Aspirin 0.65 Gm po
    Label: Aspirin 0.325 Gm/tab

20. **Order:** Gantrisin gr 8 po
    Label: Gantrisin (sulfasoxazole) 250 mg/tab

21. **Order:** Actidil 0.6 mg po
    Label: Actidil (triprolidine) 1.25 mg/5 ml

22. **Order:** Phenobarbital gr s̄s̄ po
    Label: Phenobarbital 15 mg/tab

23. **Order:** Polycillin Oral Suspension gr viis̄s̄ po
    Label: Polycillin (ampicillin) Oral Suspension 125 mg/5 ml

24. **Order:** Premarin 1.25 mg po
    Label: Premarin (estrogens conjugated) 0.625 mg/tab

25. **Order:** Thiosulfil Forte 0.25 Gm po
    Label: Thiosulfil Forte (sulfamethizole) 500 mg/tab (scored)

26. **Order:** Mebaral 0.64 Gm po
    Label: Mebaral (mephobarbital) 320 mg/tab

27. **Order:** Paradione Capsules 0.9 Gm po
    Label: Paradione (paramethadione) 300 mg/cap

28. **Order:** Nembutal Sodium gr i$\overline{ss}$ po
    Label: Nembutal Sodium (pentobarbital) 30 mg/cap

29. **Order:** Crystodigin 0.15 mg po
    Label: Crystodigin (digitoxin) 0.1 mg/tab (scored)

30. **Order:** Quinora 0.6 Gm po
    Label: Quinora (quinidine sulfate) gr iii/tab

31. **Order:** Ampicillin Suspension 500 mg po
    Label: Ampicillin Suspension 250 mg/5 ml

32. **Order:** Neg Gram Caplets 0.5 Gm po
    Label: Neg Gram (nalidixic) Caplets 500 mg/tab

33. **Order:** Tylenol gr v po
    Label: Tylenol (acetaminophen) 325 mg/tab

34. **Order:** Pen-Vee K 250 mg po
    Label: Pen-Vee K (penicillin V potassium) 125 mg/tsp
    Give _____ ml

35. **Order:** Mellaril 75 mg po
    Label: Mellaril (thioridazine) 30 mg/ml

36. **Order:** Choledyl Elixir 0.2 Gm po
    Label: Choledyl (oxtriphylline) Elixir 100 mg/5 ml

37. **Order:** Caffeine gr iii po
    Label: Caffeine 0.2 Gm/tab

38. **Order:** Chloromycetin 0.5 Gm po
    Label: Chloromycetin (chloramphenicol) 250 mg/cap

39. **Order:** Halcion 0.125 mg po
    Label: Halcion (triazolam) 0.25 mg/tab (scored)

40. **Order:** Aldomet 500 mg po
    Label: Aldomet (methyldopa) 125 mg/tab

41. **Order:** Phenergan 25 mg po
    Label: Phenergan (promethazine HCl) 12.5 mg/tab

42. **Order:** Erythromycin 0.75 Gm po
    Label: Erythromycin 250 mg/cap

43. **Order:** Robaxin 0.25 Gm po
    Label: Robaxin (methocarbamol) 500 mg/tab (scored)

44. **Order:** Quinidine Sulfate gr 6 po
    Label: Quinidine Sulfate 0.2 Gm/tab

45. **Order:** Gantrisin 2 Gm po
    Label: Gantrisin (sulfasoxizole) 500 mg/tab

46. **Order:** Nitroglycerin gr $1/600$ sublingual
    Label: Nitroglycerin 0.1 mg/tab

47. **Order:** Diuril 250 mg po
    Label: Diuril (chlorothiazide) 0.5 Gm/tab (scored)

48. **Order:** Chloral Hydrate Elixir 1.0 Gm po
    Label: Chloral Hydrate Elixir gr vii$\overline{ss}$/5 ml

49. **Order:** Lanoxin Elixir 0.03 mg po
    Label: Lanoxin (digoxin) Elixir 0.05 mg/ml

50. **Order:** Naloxone HCl 0.4 mg IM
    Label: Naloxone HCl 400 mcg (mg)/ml

51. **Order:** Pfizerpen AS 500,000 U IM
    Label: Pfizerpen AS (penicillin G procaine) 300,000 U/ml

52. **Order:** Librium 25 mg IM
    Label: Librium (chlordiazepoxide) 100 mg/2 ml

53. **Order:** Terramycin 100 mg IM
    Label: Terramycin (oxytetracycline) 250 mg/2 ml

54. **Order:** Streptomycin 500 mg IM
    Label: Streptomycin 1 Gm/2 ml

55. **Order:** Meperidine 60 mg IM
    Label: Meperidine 75 mg/1.5 ml

56. **Order:** Ergotrate 0.15 mg IM
    Label: Ergotrate (ergonovine maleate) 0.2 mg/ml
    Assume you would use a tuberculin syringe.

57. **Order:** Vitamin B_{12} 600 mcg IM
    Label: Vitamin B_{12} (cyanocobalamin) 1,000 mcg/ml

58. **Order:** Lanoxin 0.5 mg IM
    Label: Lanoxin (digoxin) 0.25 mg/ml

59. **Order:** Kantrex 500 mg IM
    Label: Kantrex (kanamycin sulfate) 1 Gm/3 ml

60. **Order:** Kanamycin Sulfate 10 mg IM
    Label: Kanamycin Sulfate 75 mg/2 ml
    Give _____ minims

61. **Order:** Vistaril 25 mg IM
    Label: Vistaril (hydroxyzine HCl) 100 mg/2 ml

62. **Order:** Digitoxin 0.05 mg IM
    Label: Digitoxin 0.2 mg/2 ml

63. **Order:** Promethazine gr 1/6 IM
    Label: Promethazine 25 mg/ml

64. **Order:** Dilaudid gr 1/64 IM
    Label: Dilaudid (hydromorphone HCl) gr 1/32/ml

65. **Order:** Lasix 40 mg IM
    Label: Lasix (furosemide) 10 mg/ml

66. **Order:** Thorazine 15 mg IM
    Label: Thorazine (chlorpromazine) 25 mg/ml

67. **Order:** Atropine Sulfate gr ¹/₁₅₀ sc
    Label: Atropine Sulfate gr ¹/₁₀₀ per ml

68. **Order:** Thorazine 35 mg IM
    Label: Thorazine (chlorpromazine) 25 mg/ml

69. **Order:** Tetracyn 100 mg IM
    Label: Tetracyn (tetracycline HCl) 250 mg/1.8 ml

70. **Order:** Meperidine 15 mg IM
    Label: Meperidine 25 mg/ml
    Give _____ minims

71. **Order:** Achromycin 0.2 Gm IM
    Label: Achromycin (tetracycline HCl) 250 mg/2 ml

72. **Order:** Kantrex 0.35 Gm IM
    Label: Kantrex (kanamycin sulfate) 0.5 Gm/ml

73. **Order:** Serpasil 2.5 mg IM
    Label: Serpasil (reserpine) 5 mg/ml

74. **Order:** Phenergan 35 mg IM
    Label: Phenergan (promethazine HCl) 50 mg/ml

75. **Order:** Kantrex 1000 mg IM
    Label: Kantrex (kanamycin sulfate) 0.5 Gm/2 ml

76. **Order:** Polycillin 0.125 Gm IM
    Label: Polycillin (ampicillin) 250 mg/1.5 ml

77. **Order:** Demerol 55 mg IM
    Label: Demerol (meperidine) 75 mg/2 ml

78. **Order:** Morphine Sulfate gr $\frac{1}{12}$ sc
    Label: Morphine Sulfate 10 mg/ml

79. **Order:** Atropine Sulfate gr $\frac{1}{150}$ IM
    Label: Atropine Sulfate 0.4 mg/ml

80. **Order:** Morphine Sulfate 10 mg IM
    Label: Morphine Sulfate gr $\frac{1}{4}$ ml
    Give _____ minims

81. **Order:** Tagamet 200 mg IM
    Label: Tagamet (cimetidine) 300 mg/2 ml in prefilled syringe
    Give _____ ml
    Discard _____ ml

82. **Order:** Terramycin 150 mg IM
    Label: Terramycin (oxytetracycline) 50 mg/ml

83. **Order:** Garamycin 50 mg IM
    Label: Garamycin (gentamicin sulfate) 80 mg/2 ml

84. **Order:** Nembutal 60 mg IM
    Label: Nembutal (pentobarbital) 100 mg/2 ml

85. **Order:** Kanamycin Sulfate 750 mg IM
    Label: Kanamycin Sulfate 1 Gm/3 ml

86. **Order:** Heparin Calcium 7,000 U sc
    Label: Heparin Calcium 10,000 U/ml
    Give _____ minims

87. **Order:** Valium 8 mg IM
    Label: Valium (diazepam) 0.1 Gm/2 ml

88. **Order:** Atropine Sulfate 0.3 mg IM
    Label: Atropine Sulfate 0.4 mg/ml

89. **Order:** Vitamin B_{12} 750 mcg IM
    Label: Vitamin B_{12} 1000 mcg/ml

90. **Order:** Folvite 1 mg IM
    Label: Folvite (folic acid) 5 mg/ml

91. **Order:** Aqua Mephyton 0.5 mg IM
    Label: Aqua Mephyton (phytonadione) 2 mg/ml

92. **Order:** Methicillin Sodium 750 mg IM
    Label: Methicillin Sodium 1 Gm dry powder
    Reconstitution: Add 1.5 ml sterile water for injection to yield 0.5
    Gm/ml.

93. **Order:** Streptomycin 400 mg IM
    Label: Streptomycin 1 Gm dry powder
    Reconstitution: Add 3.2 ml sterile water for injection to yield 250
    mg/ml.

94. **Order:** Ampicillin 350 mg IM
    Label: Ampicillin 2 Gm dry powder
    Reconstitution: Add 6.8 ml sterile water for injection to yield 250
    mg/ml.

95. **Order:** Potassium Penicillin G 40,000 U IM
    Label: Potassium Penicillin G 400,000 U dry powder
    Reconstitution: Add 4 ml sterile saline for injection to yield 100,000
    U/ml.

96. **Order:** Ampicillin 500 mg IM
    Label: Ampicillin 1 Gm dry powder
    Reconstitution: Add 2.4 ml sterile water for injection to yield 1 Gm/ 2.5 ml.

97. **Order:** Ticar 650 mg IM
    Label: Ticar (ticarcillin) 1 Gm dry powder
    Reconstitution: Add 2 ml sterile diluent to yield 1 Gm/2.6 ml.

98. **Order:** Polymyxin B 50 mg IM
    Label: Polymyxin B 150 mg dry powder
    Reconstitution: Add 2 ml sterile diluent to yield 0.075 Gm/ml.

99. **Order:** Penicillin G Potassium 750 mg IM
    Label: Penicillin G Potassium 5 Gm dry powder
    Reconstitution: Add 9.6 ml sterile diluent to yield 1 Gm/2.2 ml.

100. **Order:** Keflex 500 mg IM
     Label: Keflex 5 Gm dry powder (cephalexin) 5 Gm dry powder
     Reconstitution: Add 10 ml sterile diluent to yield 0.5 Gm/ml.

101. **Order:** Geopen 200 mg IM
     Label: Geopen (carbenicillin disodium) 1 Gm dry powder
     Reconstitution: Add 2 ml sterile water for injection to yield 1 Gm/
          2.5 ml.

102. **Order:** Mezlin 0.6 Gm IM
     Label: Mezlin (mezlocillin) 1 Gm dry powder
     Reconstitution: Add 4 ml sterile water for injection to yield 250
          mg/ml.

103. **Order:** Geopen 250 mg IM
     Label: Geopen (carbenicillin disodium) 1 Gm dry powder
     Reconstitution: Add 3.6 ml sterile water for injection to yield 1 Gm/
          4 ml.

104. **Order:** Pipracil 1200 mg IM
     Label: Pipracil (piperacillin) 2 Gm dry powder
     Reconstitution: For each gram, add 2 ml of sterile diluent to yield
     1 Gm/2.5 ml.

105. **Order:** Ampicillin 150 mg IM
     Label: Ampicillin 1 Gm dry powder
     Reconstitution: Add 3.4 ml sterile water for injection to yield 1 Gm/
     4 ml.

106. **Order:** Cefazolin Sodium 500 mg IM
     Label: Cefazolin Sodium 1 Gm dry powder
     Reconstitution: Add 3 ml sterile water for injection to yield 1 Gm/
     3 ml.

107. **Order:** Ritalin 5 mg IM
     Label: Ritalin (methylphenidate HCl) 100 mg dry powder
     Reconstitution: Add 10 ml sterile aqueous solvent to yield 100 mg/
     10 ml.

108. **Order:** BCG vaccine 400,000 U ID
     Label: BCG vaccine 8,000,000 U/ml
     Use tuberculin syringe

109. **Order:** Vitamin A 17,500 U IM
     Label: Vitamin A 50,000 U/ml

110. **Order:** Vitamin A 35,000 U IM
     Label: Vitamin A 50,000 U/ml

For 111–160, calculate flow rate in gtt/min unless directed otherwise.

111. **Order:** 3000 ml D5W IV in 24 hr
     Drop Factor: 15 gtt/ml

112. **Order:** 750 ml 5% D5NS IV in 6 hr
     Drop Factor: 15 gtt/ml

113. **Order:** 2500 ml Lactated Ringers IV in 24 hr
Drop Factor: 15 gtt/ml

114. **Order:** 1000 ml D5W IV in 4 hr
Drop Factor: 10 gtt/ml

115. **Order:** 1.5 L NS IV in 8 hr
Drop Factor: 20 gtt/ml

116. **Order:** 1000 ml Ringers Solution IV in 8 hr
Drop Factor: 15 gtt/ml

117. **Order:** 250 ml packed blood cells IV in 4 hr
Drop Factor: 10 gtt/ml

118. **Order:** 650 ml D5W in 3 hr, IV
     Drop Factor: 10 gtt/ml

119. **Order:** 1000 ml Ringers Solution IV in 8 hr
     Drop Factor: 10 gtt/ml

120. **Order:** 300 ml 10% Glucose in 8 hr, IV
     Drop Factor: 10 gtt/ml

121. **Order:** 100 ml 10% Glucose in 3 hr, IV
     Drop Factor: 15 gtt/ml

122. **Order:** 2000 ml D5W in 12 hr, IV
     Drop Factor: 10 gtt/ml

123. **Order:** 500 ml D5W in 4 hr, IV
     Drop Factor: 10 gtt/ml

124. **Order:** 1200 ml D5W in 8 hr, IV
     Drop Factor: 15 gtt/ml

125. **Order:** 900 ml NS in 6 hr, IV
     Drop Factor: 10 gtt/ml

126. **Order:** 500 ml D5W in 3.5 hr, IV
     Drop Factor: 15 gtt/ml

127. **Order:** 2000 ml of D5W in 24 hr, IV
     Drop Factor: 10 gtt/ml

128. **Order:** 500 ml Normal Saline in 12 hr, IV
Drop Factor: 60 gtt/ml

129. **Order:** 3000 ml D5W in 24 hr, IV
Drop Factor: 15 gtt/ml

130. **Order:** 1000 ml Lactated Ringers in 12 hr, IV
Drop Factor: 60 gtt/ml

131. **Order:** 750 ml Ringers Solution in 5 hr, IV
Drop Factor: 10 gtt/ml

132. **Order:** Areosporin 50 mg in 250 ml sterile water IV in 1 ½ hr
Drop Factor: 15 gtt/ml

133. **Order:** Neosporin (bacitracin) GU Irrigant 1 amp in 1000 cc Isotonic
Saline IV in 24 hr
Drop Factor: 10 gtt/ml

134. **Order:** Staphcillin (methicillin sodium) 500 mg in 50 ml NS IV at
10 ml/min
Drop Factor: 15 gtt/ml

135. **Order:** Monistat IV 200 mg diluted in 200 ml NS IV in 2 hr
Label: Monistat IV (miconazole) 200 mg/20 ml
Drop Factor: 60 gtt/ml
a. How many ml of Monistat IV should be added to the 200 ml NS?

b. What should the flow rate be?

136. **Order:** Penicillin G Potassium 15,000,000 U IV in 1000 ml D5W
to infuse over 24 hr
Label: Penicillin G Potassium 20,000,000 U
Reconstitution: Dilute with 31.6 ml of D5W to yield 500,000 U/ml.
Drop Factor: 15 gtt/ml
a. How much should be added to the 1000 ml of D5W?

b. What should the flow rate be?

137. **Order:** 2500 ml D5W IV
Drop Factor: 10 gtt/ml
Flow Rate: 40 gtt/min
How long should it take the IV to infuse?

138. **Order:** Zovirax 5 mg/kg IVPB in 100 ml D5W in 60 min
Weight: 70 kg
Label: Zovirax (acyclovir) 500 mg dry powder
Drop Factor: 60 gtt/ml
Directions: Reconstitute by adding 10 ml sterile diluent to yield 50 mg/ml.
a. How many ml of reconstituted Zovirax should be added to the 100 ml D5W?

b. What should the flow rate be?

139. **Order:** Aminophylline 1 Gm in 1000 ml D5½NS IV to infuse at 35 mg/hr
Drop Factor: 60 gtt/ml
What should the flow rate be?

140. **Order:** Mefoxin 2 Gm IVPB in 100 ml Sodium Chloride 0.9% in
           60 min
     Label: Mefoxin (cefoxitan sodium) 1 Gm dry powder
     Reconstitution: Dilute with 10 ml sterile water for injection to yield
           1 Gm/10.5 ml.
     Drop Factor: 15 gtt/ml
     a. How many ml Mefoxin should be added to the IV solution?

     b. What should the flow rate be?

141. **Order:** Cefazolin Sodium 1 Gm in 100 ml 10% DW IV to infuse in
           60 min via Volutrol
     Label: Cefazolin Sodium 1 Gm dry powder
     Reconstitution: Dilute with 2.5 ml sterile water for injection to yield
           1 Gm/3 ml.
     Drop Factor: 60 gtt/ml
     What should the flow rate be?

142. **Order:** Heparin Sodium 30,000 U in 250 ml D5W IV to infuse at
           10 ml/hr (via IV pump)
     Label: Heparin Sodium 20,000 U/ml
     Drop Factor: 60 gtt/ml
     a. How many ml of Heparin should be added to the IV solution?

b. What should the flow rate be?

143. **Order:** Heparin Sodium 10,000 U in 100 ml D5W IV to infuse at
     1,200 U/hr
     Label: Heparin Sodium 10,000 U/ml
     Drop Factor: 60 gtt/ml
     a. What should the flow rate be?

    b. How many hours will it take to complete the IV?

144. **Order:** Regular Insulin 10 U/hr IV in 500 ml NS to infuse in 6 hr
     Label: Regular Insulin 100 U/ml
     How many units of Insulin should be added to the IV solution in
     order to administer the Insulin over a period of 6 hrs?

145. **Order:** Lidocaine HCl 1 Gm in 250 ml D5W (IV mini-bottle/saline
     lock) to infuse at a rate of 2 mg/min
     Label: Lidocaine HCl 1 Gm/5 ml
     Drop Factor: 60 gtt/ml
     What should the flow rate be?

146. **Order:** Dopamine HCl 400 mg in 500 ml D5W to infuse at 5 mcg/kg/min IV

     Weight: 75 kg

     Drop Factor: 60 gtt/ml

     a. How many mcg/min should be administered?

     b. How many ml/hr will provide the required dose?

     c. How many gtt/min will provide the required dose?

     d. How many mcg/gtt will be administered?

147. **Order:** Heparin Sodium 7,000 U in 250 ml D5W at 0.4 U/kg/min IV

     Weight: 129 lb

     Drop Factor: 60 gtt/ml

     a. How many U/min should be administered?

b. How many ml/hr will provide the required dose?

c. How many gtt/min will provide the required dose?

148. **Order:** Nipride (nitroprusside sodium) 50 mg in 250 ml D5W at 4
     mcg/kg/min IV
     Weight: 77.6 kg
     Drop Factor: 60 gtt/ml
     a. How many mcg/min should be administered?

b. How many ml/hr will provide the required dose?

c. How many gtt/min will provide the required dose?

d. How many mcg/gtt will be administered?

149. **Order:** Dobutamine HCl 250 mg in 500 ml 5% Dextrose in Lactated
Ringers at 10 mcg/kg/min IV
Weight: 181 lb
Drop Factor: 60 gtt/ml
a. How many mcg/min should be administered?

b. How many ml/hr will provide the required dose?

c. How many gtt/min will provide the required dose?

d. How many mcg/gtt will be administered?

150. **Order:** Intropin (dopamine HCl) 400 mg in 500 ml D5W at 10 mcg/
kg/min IV
Weight: 88.6 kg
Drop Factor: 60 gtt/ml
a. How many mcg/min should be administered?

b. How many ml/hr will provide the required dose?

c. How many gtt/min will provide the required dose?

d. How many mcg/gtt will be administered?

151. **Order:** Nitroprusside Sodium 50 mg in 250 ml D5W at 4 mcg/kg/
       min IV
     Weight: 109 lb
     Drop Factor: 60 gtt/ml
     a. How many mcg/min should be administered?

b. How many ml/hr will provide the required dose?

c. How many gtt/min will provide the required dose?

d. How many mcg/gtt will be administered?

152. **Order:** Infuse Nitroprusside Sodium 50 mg in 250 ml D5W. Titrate
0.5–1.5 mcg/kg/min to maintain the systolic blood pressure
below 140 mm Hg.
Weight: 198 lb

a. What is the concentration of the solution in mcg/ml?

b. How many mcg/min will administer the ordered range of titration?
Lower (0.5 mcg/kg/min):

Upper (1.5 mcg/kg/min):

c. How many ml/hr or gtt/min will administer the ordered range of titration?
Lower:

Upper:

d. What is the titration (concentration) factor in mcg/gtt?

e. The present systolic blood pressure reading is 155 mm Hg. Increase the gtt/min by 5 gtt. How many mcg/min will the patient now be receiving?

153. **Order:** Heparin Sodium 25,000 U in 500 ml D5W IV to infuse over 24 hr via IV pump
To how many ml/hr should the IV pump be set?

154. **Order:** Penicillin G Potassium 8 million units IVPB in 100 ml D5W
to infuse over 1 hr
Label: Penicillin G Potassium 20,000,000 U dry powder
Reconstitution: Add 11.5 ml sterile water for injection to yield
1,000,000 U/ml.
Drop Factor: 15 gtt/ml
a. How many ml of reconstituted solution should be added to 100
ml D5W?

b. What should the flow rate be?

155. **Order:** KCl 40 mEq in 1000 ml D5W IV
Drop Factor: 15 gtt/ml
Flow Rate: 35 gtt/min
How long should it take the IV to infuse?

156. **Order:** Aminophylline 150 mg IVPB in 100 ml D5W to infuse in
60 min
Label: Aminophylline 250 mg/10 ml
Drop Factor: 60 gtt/ml
a. How many ml should be added to the 100 ml D5W?

b. What should the flow rate be?

157. **Order:** Zovirax (acyclovir) 5 mg/kg IVPB in 100 ml D5W to infuse in 60 min
     Label: Zovirax 500 mg dry powder
     Weight: 130 lb
     Reconstitution: Add 10 ml sterile water for injection to yield 500 mg/10 ml.
     Drop Factor: 60 gtt/ml
     a. How many ml should be added to the 100 ml D5W?

     b. What should the flow rate be?

158. **Order:** Achromycin 500 mg IVPB in 100 ml D5W to infuse in 1 hr
     Label: Achromycin (tetracycline HCl) 0.5 Gm dry powder
     Reconstitution: Add 10 ml sterile diluent to yield 250 mg per 5 ml.
     Drop Factor: 15 gtt/ml
     a. How many ml of reconstituted solution should be added to 100 ml D5W?

     b. What should the flow rate be?

159. **Order:** Vistaril (hydroxyzine HCl) 75 mg in 100 ml NS IV via Met-
    riset
    Drop Factor: 60 gtt/ml
    Flow Rate: 100 gtt/min
    How long should it take the IV to infuse?

160. **Order:** 1000 ml D5½NS IV via central venous catheter to infuse
    at 150 ml/hr for first 500 ml. Add MVI 10 ml to remaining
    500 ml and continue infusion at 75 ml/hr. Use an IV pump.
    Label: MVI 10 ml/ampule
    Drop Factor: 60 gtt/ml
    a. What should the flow rate be for the first 500 ml?

    b. To what should the flow rate be adjusted for the remaining
       500 ml?

161. **Order:** Heparin Sodium 10,000 U in 100 ml D5W IV to infuse at
    10 gtt/min
    Drop Factor: 60 gtt/ml
    How many units of Heparin is the patient receiving in 24 hours?

162. **Order:** Digoxin 0.375 mg IV Push at a rate of 0.5 ml/min
     Label: Digoxin 0.25 mg/ml
     a. How many ml of Digoxin should be administered?

     b. How long should it take to administer the IV Digoxin?

163. **Order:** Lidocaine HCl 1 mg/kg via IV Push
     Weight: 154 lb
     How many mg should be administered per dose?

164. **Order:** Adriamycin 30 mg/M^2 via IV bolus at a rate of 3 mg/min
     BSA = 0.5 M^2
     Label: Adriamycin (doxorubicin HCl) 10 mg. Dilute in 5 ml sodium
     chloride for injection.
     a. How many ml should be administered per dose?

     b. How long should it take to inject the Adriamycin?

165. **Order:** Valium 0.3 mg/kg via IV bolus at a rate of 5 mg/min
     Label: Valium (diazepam) 5 mg/ml
     Weight: 40 lb
     a. How many ml of Valium should the child receive per dose?

     b. How long should it take to inject the Valium?

166. **Order:** Lorfan 0.02 mg/kg of body weight via IV push at a rate of
                1 mg/min
     Label: Lorfan (levallorphan tartrate) 0.4 mg/ml
     Weight: 35 lb
     a. How many ml Lorfan should the child receive per dose?

     b. How long should it take to inject the Lorfan?

167. **Order:** TPN 1000 ml Liposyn II 20% IV
     How many kcal of fat are provided?

168. **Order:** CPN 1000 ml 5% dextrose in 0.9% Sodium Chloride IV
     How many kcal of carbohydrate are provided?

169. **Order:** PTPN 500 ml Aminosyn II 3.5% IV
     How many kcal of protein are provided?

170. **Order:** Hyperalimentation 1500 ml Liposyn 10% IV
     How many kcal of fat are provided?

171. **Order:** Methimazole 0.4 mg/kg po in three divided doses
     Label: Methimazole 5 mg/tab (scored)
     Weight: 79 lb

172. **Order:** Valproic Acid 5 mg/kg po in three divided doses
     Label: Valproic Acid 250 mg/5 ml
     Weight: 165 lb

173. **Order:** Isoniazid 5 mg/kg po
     Label: Isoniazid 100 mg/tab
     Weight: 60 kg

174. **Order:** Sus-Phrine 0.005 ml/kg sc
     Label: Sus-Phrine (epinephrine) 2.5 mg/5 ml
     Weight: 44 lb

175. **Order:** Paromomycin 25 mg/kg/day po in three divided doses
     Label: Paromomycin 250 mg/capsule
     Weight: 160 lb
     How many capsules should be administered/dose?

176. **Order:** Symmetrel Syrup 8.8 mg/kg po in two divided doses
     Label: Symmetrel (amantadine) Syrup 50 mg/5 ml
     Weight: 35 lb

177. **Order:** Terramycin 3 mg/lb/day in two divided doses IM
Label: Terramycin (oxytetracycline) 100 mg/2 ml
Weight: 20 lb

178. **Order:** Kantrex 15 mg/kg/day in two divided doses IM
Label: Kantrex (kanamycin sulfate) 75 mg/2 ml
Weight: 55 lb

179. **Order:** Vibramycin 2 mg/lb in two divided doses po
Label: Vibramycin Calcium Syrup (doxycycline calcium oral suspension) 50 mg/5 ml
Weight: 38 kg

180. **Order:** Tetracyn Syrup 50 mg/kg/day in four divided doses po
Label: Tetracyn (tetracycline HCl) Syrup 125 mg/tsp
Weight: 60 lb
Give _____ ml/dose

181. **Order:** Achromycin 10 mg/kg/day in two divided doses IM
     Label: Achromycin (tetracycline HCl) 100 mg/2 ml
     Weight: 12 lb

182. **Order:** Dobutrex 250 mg in 500 ml 5% Dextrose IV at 5 mcg (μg)/
     kg/min
     Label: Dobutrex (dobutamine HCl) 250 mg/20 ml
     Weight: 143 lb

183. **Order:** Rondomycin Syrup 6 mg/lb/day in four divided doses po
     Label: Rondomycin (methacycline) Syrup 75 mg/5 ml
     Weight: 62 lb

184. **Order:** Kefzol 25 mg/kg/day in four divided doses IM
     Label: Kefzol (cefazolin sodium) 250 mg dry powder
     Weight: 30 lb
     Reconstitution: Dilute in 2 ml sterile water for injection to yield
     125 mg/ml.

185. **Order:** Acetaminophen Elixir 10 mg/kg/dose po
     Label: Acetaminophen Elixir 160 mg/5 ml
     Weight: 54 lb

For 186–190, use the West nomogram and label factor method.

186. Child's height: 33 in
     Child's weight: 28 lb
     Adult dose: Dilantin (phenytoin sodium) 100 mg
     Find the child's dose.

187. Child's height: 95 cm
     Child's weight: 15 kg
     Adult dose: Lomotil (diphenoxylate HCl and atropine sulfate) 5 ml
     Find the child's dose.

188. Child's height: 104 cm
     Child's weight: 17 kg
     Adult dose: Atropine Sulfate 0.4 mg
     Find the child's dose.

189. Child's height: 52 in
     Child's weight: 50 lb
     Adult dose: Digoxin 0.125 mg
     Find the child's dose.

190. Child's height: 58.5 cm
     Child's weight: 5.9 kg
     Adult dose: Valium (diazepam) 2 mg
     Find the child's dose.

For 191–200, use the drug labels in Figure 13-1 and calculate the correct dosage.

191. **Order:** Ticar (ticarcillin) 250 mg IM

192. **Order:** Carbenicillin Disodium 4 Gm IV

193. **Order:** Vasopressin 8 Units sc

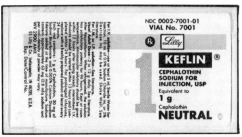

a.

NDC 0002-7001-01
VIAL No. 7001
Rx Lilly
KEFLIN®
CEPHALOTHIN
SODIUM FOR
INJECTION, USP
Equivalent to
1 g
Cephalothin
NEUTRAL

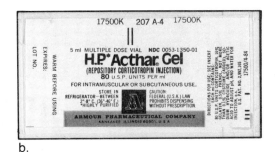

b.

17500K   207 A-4   17500K
5 ml MULTIPLE DOSE VIAL NDC 0053-1350-01
H.P.® Acthar® Gel
(REPOSITORY CORTICOTROPIN INJECTION)
80 U.S.P. UNITS PER ml
FOR INTRAMUSCULAR OR SUBCUTANEOUS USE.
STORE IN
REFRIGERATOR—BETWEEN
2°-8°C (36°-46°F)
"HIGHLY PURIFIED"
CAUTION:
FEDERAL (U.S.A.) LAW
PROHIBITS DISPENSING
WITHOUT PRESCRIPTION.
ARMOUR PHARMACEUTICAL COMPANY
KANKAKEE ILLINOIS 60901, U S A

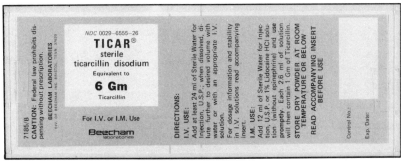

c.

NDC 0029-6555-26
TICAR®
sterile
ticarcillin disodium
Equivalent to
6 Gm
Ticarcillin
For I.V. or I.M. Use
Beecham
laboratories

CAUTION: Federal law prohibits dispensing without prescription.
BEECHAM LABORATORIES
DIV. OF BEECHAM INC. BRISTOL TENN. 37620
7185/B

DIRECTIONS:
I.V. USE:
Add at least 24 ml of Sterile Water for Injection, U.S.P. when dissolved, dilute further to desired volume with water or with an appropriate I.V. solution.
For dosage information and stability in I.V. solutions read accompanying insert.
I.M. USE:
Add 12 ml of Sterile Water for Injection, U.S.P. or 1% Lidocaine HCl solution (without epinephrine) and use promptly. Each 2.6 ml of solution will then contain 1 Gm of Ticarcillin.
STORE DRY POWDER AT ROOM TEMPERATURE OR BELOW
READ ACCOMPANYING INSERT BEFORE USE

Control No.:
Exp. Date:

d.

LyphoMed®
POTASSIUM
CHLORIDE
INJECTION, USP
(2 mEq/mL)
40 mEq
20 mL
Multiple Dose Vial

N 0469-2067-15 Sterile. Nonpyrogenic. 967-20
MUST BE DILUTED PRIOR TO IV ADMINISTRATION
Each mL contains: Potassium Chloride 149 mg;
Methylparaben 0.05%; Propylparaben 0.005%;
Water for Injection q.s. pH adjusted with HCl or
KOH if necessary. 4000 mOsmol/L.
Usual Dose: See Package Insert.
LyphoMed, Inc., Rosemont, IL 60018   B-87

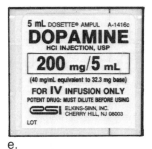

e.

5 mL DOSETTE® AMPUL   A-1416c
DOPAMINE
HCl INJECTION, USP
200 mg/5 mL
(40 mg/mL equivalent to 32.3 mg base)
FOR IV INFUSION ONLY
POTENT DRUG; MUST DILUTE BEFORE USING
esi ELKINS-SINN, INC.
CHERRY HILL, NJ 08003
LOT

f.

LOT
EXP.   To open—Cut seal along dotted line.
25 DOSETTE® VIALS—Each contains 1 mL   NDC 0641-0140-25
MEPERIDINE
HCl INJECTION, USP
50 mg/mL
FOR INTRAMUSCULAR,
SUBCUTANEOUS OR
SLOW INTRAVENOUS USE
WARNING: May be habit forming.

Each mL contains meperidine hydrochloride 50 mg, sodium metabisulfite 1.5 mg and phenol 5 mg in Water for Injection. Buffered with acetic acid-sodium acetate. pH 3.5-6.0. Sealed under nitrogen.
USUAL DOSE—See package insert.
Do not use if precipitated.
Store at controlled room temperature 15°-30°C (59°-86°F).
CAUTION: Federal law prohibits dispensing without prescription.
Product Code
0140-25   B-50140g

esi ELKINS-SINN, INC. Cherry Hill, NJ 08003-4099
A subsidiary of A. H. Robins Company

g.

QUAD
NDC 51309-930-01
Vasopressin
Injection, USP
Synthetic
10 Units
0.5 mL
For IM or SC
Use Only
0.5 mL
Multiple Dose Vial
QUAD Pharmaceuticals
Indianapolis, IN 46268, U.S.A.
L-02-149

Figure 13-1 (*Part a Courtesy Eli Lilly & Co.; Part b Courtesy Armour Pharmaceutical Company; Part c Courtesy Beecham Laboratories; Part d Courtesy LyphoMed, Inc.; Parts e, f, i, and k Courtesy Elkins-Sinn, Inc., A Subsidiary of A. H. Robins Company; Part g Courtesy QUAD Pharmaceuticals; Parts h and l Courtesy Roerig, A Division of Pfizer Inc.; Part j Courtesy Marion Laboratories, Inc.; Part m Courtesy Boehringer Ingelheim Pharmaceuticals, Inc.*)

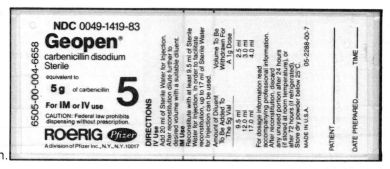

h.

NDC 0049-1419-83

Geopen®

carbenicillin disodium
Sterile

equivalent to

5 g of carbenicillin

5

For IM or IV use

CAUTION: Federal law prohibits dispensing without prescription.

ROERIG *Pfizer*

A division of Pfizer Inc., N.Y., N.Y. 10017

6505-00-004-6658

DIRECTIONS

IV Use
Add 20 ml of Sterile Water for Injection to the vial. After reconstitution dilute further to desired volume with a suitable diluent.

IM Use
Reconstitute with at least 9.5 ml of Sterile Water for Injection. In order to facilitate reconstitution, up to 17 ml of Sterile Water for Injection can be used.

Amount of Diluent To Be Added To The 5g Vial	Volume To Be Withdrawn For A 1g Dose
9.5 ml	2.5 ml
12.0 ml	3.0 ml
17.0 ml	4.0 ml

For dosage information read accompanying professional information. After reconstitution, discard any unused portion after 24 hours (if stored at room temperature), or after 72 hours (if refrigerated). Store dry powder below 25°C.

MADE IN U.S.A.

05-2288-00-7

PATIENT _____ TIME _____

DATE PREPARED _____

---

i.

10 ml SINGLE USE VIAL
NDC 0641-2205-41

AMINOPHYLLINE

INJECTION, USP

250 mg/10 ml

(25 mg/ml)

FOR SLOW INTRAVENOUS USE

NO PRESERVATIVE

Each ml contains amino-phylline anhydrous 25 mg (anhydrous theophylline 19.7 mg and ethylenediamine 5.3 mg). Additional ethylenediamine may have been used to adjust pH to 8.6-9.0. Sealed under nitrogen.

Note: Do not use if crystals have separated. Store at controlled room temperature 15° to 30°C (59° to 86°F).

PROTECT FROM LIGHT

Caution: Federal law prohibits dispensing without prescription.

SINGLE USE: DESTROY UNUSED CONTENTS

Usual Dose: See package insert for complete prescribing information.

A-2205

Product Code
2205-41

LOT   EXP

esi ELKINS-SINN, INC. Cherry Hill, NJ 08034

A subsidiary of A. H. Robins Company

---

j.

6505-00-527-8960   NDC 0088-1550-41

NITRO-BID® 2.5

(nitroglycerin)

EACH CONTROLLED-RELEASE CAPSULE CONTAINS:

Nitroglycerin . . . . 2.5 mg

DOSAGE: One capsule two or three times daily, at 8- to 12-hour intervals. Refer to package insert for full prescribing information.

CAUTION: Federal law prohibits dispensing without prescription.

KEEP OUT OF REACH OF CHILDREN

PHARMACIST: Store at a controlled room temperature (59°-86°F).

Dispense only in original unopened container.

SPECIMEN COPY

PHARMACEUTICAL DIVISION
M MARION LABORATORIES, INC.
KANSAS CITY, MISSOURI 64137

E7

60 Plateau CAPS®

---

k.

10 ml Multiple Dose Vial
NDC 0641-2460-41

HEPARIN

SODIUM INJECTION, USP

5000 USP units/ml

FOR IV OR SC USE

Usual Dose: See enclosed insert for complete prescribing information.

Each ml contains heparin sodium 5000 USP units and sodium chloride 7 mg yet Water for Injection with 0.01 ml benzyl alcohol, pH may be adjusted (Acid or Alkali) with sodium hydroxide and/or hydrochloric acid to 5.0 - 7.5.

DERIVED FROM PORCINE INTESTINES

Caution: Federal law prohibits dispensing without prescription.

A-2460c

Product Code 2460-41

LOT   EXP.

esi ELKINS-SINN, INC. Cherry Hill, NJ 08034

A subsidiary of A. H. Robins Company

---

l.

10 ml Vial

Terramycin®

oxytetracycline
INTRAMUSCULAR SOLUTION®
50 mg/ml

contains 2% lidocaine

CAUTION: Federal law prohibits dispensing without prescription.

ROERIG *Pfizer*

A division of Pfizer Inc., N.Y., N.Y. 10017

Each ml contains (w/v) 50 mg oxytetracycline, 2% lidocaine, 2.5% magnesium chloride hexahydrate, 0.1% formaldehyde sulfoxylate, 1% monoethanolamine, 2.5% monoethanolamide, 0.02% propyl gallate, 1% citric acid, 4.1%, propylene glycol and 16.5% water.

RECOMMENDED STORE BELOW 86°F (30°C)

For Intramuscular use only

READ ACCOMPANYING PROFESSIONAL INFORMATION

DOSAGE:
ADULTS: The usual daily dose 250 mg administered once every 24 hours or 300 mg given in divided doses at 12 hour intervals.
CHILDREN ABOVE EIGHT YEARS OF AGE: 15-25 mg/kg body weight up to a maximum of 250 mg per single daily injection. Dosage may be divided and given at 8 to 12 hour intervals.

*U.S. Pat. Nos. 3,017,323 and 3,026,248

MADE IN U.S.A.

---

m.

Boehringer Ingelheim Pharmaceuticals, Inc. Ridgefield, CT 06877
Licensed from Boehringer Ingelheim International GmbH

Alupent®

(metaproterenol sulfate USP)

Syrup   10 ml

METABISULFITE FREE

Professional sample

Boehringer Ingelheim

Each teaspoonful (5 ml) contains metaproterenol sulfate, 10 mg.

Dosage: Children: 6-9 yrs or under 60 lbs, 1 tsp 3 or 4 times daily. Over 9 yrs or over 60 lbs, 2 tsp 3 or 4 times daily. Adults: 2 tsp 3 or 4 times daily.

Read accompanying prescribing information for full details.

Caution: Federal law prohibits dispensing without prescription.

Store below 86°F (30°C). Protect from light.

826592

Figure 13-1   Cont.

194. **Order:** Heparin Sodium 3000 U sc

195. **Order:** Potassium Chloride 30 mEq IV

196. **Order:** Demerol (meperidine) 35 mg IM

197. **Order:** Aminophylline 150 mg IV

198. **Order:** Oxytetracycline 100 mg IM

199. **Order:** Dopamine HCl 125 mg IV

200. **Order:** H. P. Acthar Gel (corticotropin) 70 U IM

201. The patient is to receive Demerol 75 mg and Phenergan 12.5 mg IM in the same syringe.
     Label: Demerol (meperidine hydrochloride) 50 mg/ml
     Phenergan (promethazine hydrochloride) 25 mg/ml
     How many ml would contain the total amount of medication ordered?

202. A child weighing 35 lb is to receive Monistat i.v. (miconazole) 15 mg/kg IV q 8 hr. How many mg of Monistat will be administered in 24 hrs?

203. The patient is to receive Tagamet 800 mg per day to be divided in equal doses and given q 6 hr.
     Label: Tagamet (cimetidine hydrochloride) 300 mg/2 ml
     How many ml should be administered per dose?

204. The patient is to receive 125 ml/hr of 0.9% NS IV. How many ml/min will be administered?

205. The patient is to receive Lipo-Hepin 8,000 units sc.
     Label: Lipo-Hepin (heparin sodium) 10,000 U/ml
     How many ml should be given?

206. An infant weighing 20 lb is to receive Gantricin 75 mg/kg/day in 6
     divided doses po.
     Label: Gantricin (sulfisoxazole) 0.5 Gm/tsp
     How many ml should be given per dose?

207. The patient is to receive 1000 ml 5% D/W IV. How many Gm of
     glucose does the solution contain?

208. The patient has an IV of 1000 ml D5W to which Potassium Chloride
     10 mEq is to be added.
     Label: Potassium Chloride 2 mEq/ml
     How many ml of KCl should be added to the IV solution?

209. The patient is to receive Pitocin (oxytocin) 5 units in 500 ml Ringer's
     lactate solution IV. How many milliunits (mU) of Pitocin does one
     ml of the solution contain?

210. The patient is to receive NegGram Suspension 2 Gm per day po in equal doses q 6 hr.
Label: NegGram (naladaxic acid) 250 mg/tsp
How many ml should each dose contain?

211. The patient is to receive 500 ml of 25% D/W. How many kcal of Dextrose would the patient be receiving?

212. A patient weighing 160 lb is to receive Dobutrex (dobutamine hydrochloride) 7.5 mcg (μg)/kg/min IV. How many μg/hr will the patient receive?

213. The patient is to receive 750 ml of 5% D/NS in 5 hours. How many ml/hr should the patient receive?

214. A patient receives a total daily dosage of 2 Gm Chloromycetin po in equal doses q 6 hr.
Label: Chloromycetin (chloramphenicol) 250 mg/cap
How many capsules should the patient receive per dose?

215. The patient is to receive Revimine (dopamine hydrochloride) 400 mg in 1000 ml D5W IV to be administered at a rate of 5 mcg/kg/min.
How many mcg of Revimine does 1 ml of solution contain?

216. A patient weighing 150 lb is to receive Dopastat (dopamine hydrochloride) 400 mg in 500 ml of IV solution to be administered at a rate of 5 mcg/kg/min. How many ml/hr should the patient receive?

217. The patient is to receive Ritodrine Hydrochloride 150 mg in 500 ml of 5% Dextrose solution to infuse at a rate of 0.2 mg/min. How many ml/hr should be administered to infuse the ordered dose?

218. A child weighing 75 lb is to receive Morphine Sulfate 0.1 mg/kg of body weight sc.
Label: Morphine Sulfate 5 mg/ml
How many ml should be administered?

219. The patient is to receive Kefzol (cefazolin sodium) 8 Gm IM in 24 hrs to be given in equal doses at 6 hr intervals. How many mg should be administered per dose?

220. The patient is receiving an IV to which a piggyback of 100 ml of medication is to be added. The IVPB is to be infused in 45 min.
Drop Factor: 60 microdrops/ml
How many microdrops will be administered/min?

(*Note:* See Appendix C for answer key.)

Arithmetic Review

··

Roman Numerals

A. Express the following Arabic numerals as Roman numerals.

1. 6		6. 46	
2. 50		7. 17	
3. 3		8. 38	
4. 12		9. 25	
5. 24		10. 9	

B. Express the following Roman numerals as Arabic numerals.

1. XLVII		6. VII	
2. XXIX		7. II	
3. V		8. LXVI	
4. CXII		9. CCCIX	
5. MCMXXXIII		10. XIII	

Addition

Add the following whole numbers.

1. 12 +16	4. 28 48 +69	6. 642 91 +357	8. 81 648 + 43
2. 22 + 3	5. 39 88 +16	7. 611 292 +386	9. 8397 184 +5240
3. 43 +15			

10.   31,017
          13
     + 2,377

11. 6 + 23 =

12. 13 + 52 =

13. 19 + 32 + 15 =

14. 17 + 231 + 92 =

15. 700 + 26 + 845 =

16. 9 + 47 + 299 =

17. 393 + 209 + 567 =

18. 2,091 + 581 + 6,727 =

19. 8 + 5,496 + 745 =

20. 40 + 50,008 + 9,833 =

Subtraction

Subtract the following whole numbers.

1.   29
     − 6

2.   215
     − 38

3.   5309
     − 342

4.   7333
     −4281

5.   73
     −41

6.   303
     − 55

7.   12,965
     −   492

8.   138
     − 25

9.   8846
     −8721

10.   965
      − 82

11. 42 − 31 =

12. 54 − 36 =

13. 235 − 66 =

14. 465 − 203 =

15. 209 − 65 =

16. 6699 − 301 =

17. 1124 − 908 =

18. 1865 − 1392 =

19. 32,945 − 2,030 =

20. 56,841 − 32,931 =

Multiplication

Multiply the following numbers.

1.   8
     ×4

2.   24
     ×13

3.   311
     ×252

4.   15
     × 9

5.   143
     × 91

6.   609
     × 23

7.   497
     ×704

8.   2536
     × 219

9.   1551
     × 69

10.   733
      ×300

11. 19 × 4 =

12. 21 × 6 =

13. 34 × 12 =

14. 62 × 18 =

15. 256 × 79 =

16. 689 × 203 =

17. 181 × 117 =

18. 1598 × 200 =

19. 18,452 × 1,501 =

20. 986 × 1000 =

Division

Solve the following division problems. Carry answers to two decimal places and round to nearest tenth.

1. $4\overline{)20}$
2. $25\overline{)295}$
3. $8\overline{)164}$
4. $3\overline{)925}$
5. $13\overline{)2363}$

6. $16\overline{)5493}$
7. $232\overline{)2696}$
8. $473\overline{)9652}$
9. $281\overline{)6795}$
10. $596\overline{)9235}$

11. $105 \div 5 =$
12. $648 \div 8 =$
13. $2222 \div 11 =$
14. $6950 \div 30 =$
15. $6393 \div 16 =$

16. $15,321 \div 35 =$
17. $16,209 \div 10 =$
18. $18,492 \div 933 =$
19. $802,495 \div 436 =$
20. $111,666 \div 606 =$

Fractions

A. Reduce the following fractions to lowest terms.

> **Rule:** Divide both numerator and denominator by the largest whole number that will go evenly into each.

Example: $\dfrac{5}{10} = \dfrac{5 \div 5}{10 \div 5} = \dfrac{1}{2}$

Practice:

1. $\dfrac{2}{6}$
2. $\dfrac{3}{9}$
3. $\dfrac{4}{8}$
4. $\dfrac{3}{15}$
5. $\dfrac{5}{55}$

6. $\dfrac{12}{48}$
7. $\dfrac{9}{10}$
8. $\dfrac{14}{56}$
9. $\dfrac{18}{80}$
10. $\dfrac{255}{1530}$

B. Convert the following mixed numbers to improper fractions.

> **Rule:** Multiply the whole number by the denominator, add to numerator, and place this sum over the original denominator.

Example: $5\dfrac{3}{8} = 5 \times 8 = 40 + 3 = \dfrac{43}{8}$

Practice:

1. 2 ¾   6. 9 ⅖

2. 7 ⁸⁄₉   7. 1 ⅔

3. 5 ³⁄₁₀   8. 1 ½

4. 12 ¼   9. 10 ⅖

5. 6 ⅔   10. 8 ³⁄₆

C. Convert the following improper fractions to mixed numbers. Reduce the fraction to lowest terms.

> **Rule:** Divide the denominator into the numerator and reduce to lowest terms.

Example: $\dfrac{72}{9} = 72 \div 9 = 8$

$\qquad\dfrac{45}{6} = 45 \div 6 = 7\dfrac{3}{6} = 7\dfrac{1}{2}$

Practice:

1. $\dfrac{25}{6}$ 4. $\dfrac{62}{8}$ 7. $\dfrac{122}{9}$ 10. $\dfrac{99}{2}$

2. $\dfrac{19}{3}$ 5. $\dfrac{16}{11}$ 8. $\dfrac{125}{23}$

3. $\dfrac{94}{5}$ 6. $\dfrac{40}{13}$ 9. $\dfrac{82}{4}$

D. Add the following fractions. Convert answer to mixed numbers when possible and reduce fraction to lowest terms.

> **Rule:** When the denominators are the same, add the numerators and place this sum over the original denominator.

Example:
$$\begin{array}{r} \dfrac{1}{8} \\[4pt] +\dfrac{3}{8} \\[4pt] \hline \dfrac{4}{8} = \dfrac{1}{2} \end{array}$$

> **Rule:** 1. When the denominators are not the same, determine the least common denominator (LCD) by finding the smallest number divisible by both denominators.
> 2. Divide each denominator by this LCD and multiply each numerator by its respective quotient.
> 3. Add the numerators, place over the LCD and reduce to lowest terms.

Examples:

$$\frac{2}{16} = \frac{2}{16}$$
$$+\frac{1}{8} = +\frac{2}{16}$$
$$\frac{4}{16} = \frac{1}{4}$$

LCD = 16

$$\frac{7}{10} = \frac{49}{70}$$
$$+\frac{9}{35} = +\frac{18}{70}$$
$$\frac{67}{70}$$

LCD = 70

Practice:

1. $\dfrac{7}{9}$
$+\dfrac{4}{9}$

2. $\dfrac{3}{4}$
$+\dfrac{1}{4}$

3. $\dfrac{2}{6}$
$+\dfrac{5}{6}$

4. $\dfrac{1}{12}$
$+\dfrac{4}{12}$

5. $\dfrac{1}{15}$
$\dfrac{2}{15}$
$+\dfrac{6}{15}$

6. $\dfrac{32}{90}$
$+\dfrac{16}{90}$

7. $\dfrac{1}{3}$
$+\dfrac{3}{4}$

8. $\dfrac{2}{5}$
$\dfrac{6}{10}$
$+\dfrac{3}{5}$

9. $\dfrac{2}{3}$
$\dfrac{5}{6}$
$+\dfrac{4}{6}$

10. $\dfrac{60}{48}$
$+\dfrac{34}{48}$

11. $\dfrac{1}{2} + \dfrac{2}{2} =$

12. $\dfrac{2}{3} + \dfrac{1}{3} =$

13. $\dfrac{5}{8} + \dfrac{2}{8} =$

14. $\dfrac{2}{3} + \dfrac{1}{4} + \dfrac{5}{6} =$

15. $\dfrac{2}{12} + \dfrac{3}{18} + \dfrac{2}{2} =$

16. $\dfrac{2}{3} + \dfrac{5}{12} + \dfrac{2}{4} =$

17. $\dfrac{3}{15} + \dfrac{10}{60} + \dfrac{1}{12} =$

18. $\dfrac{1}{4} + \dfrac{16}{64} + \dfrac{8}{32} =$

19. $\dfrac{9}{10} + \dfrac{20}{100} + \dfrac{6}{10} =$

20. $\dfrac{32}{18} + \dfrac{1}{18} + \dfrac{9}{72} =$

E. Subtract the following fractions. Convert answer to mixed numbers when possible and reduce fraction to lowest terms.

Rule: When the denominators are the same, subtract the numerators and place this difference over the original denominator.

Example:

$$\frac{7}{10}$$
$$-\frac{3}{10}$$
$$\frac{4}{10} = \frac{2}{5}$$

Rule: 1. When the denominators are not the same, determine the least common denominator (LCD) by finding the smallest number divisible by both denominators.
2. Divide each denominator by this LCD and multiply each numerator by its respective quotient.
3. Subtract the numerators, place over the LCD and reduce to lowest terms.

Example:

$$\frac{13}{21}$$
$$-\frac{4}{21}$$
$$\frac{9}{21} = \frac{3}{7}$$

Practice:

1. $\frac{5}{6}$
    $-\frac{1}{6}$

2. $\frac{3}{7}$
    $-\frac{2}{7}$

3. $\frac{7}{14}$
    $-\frac{3}{14}$

4. $\frac{3}{4}$
    $-\frac{2}{4}$

5. $\frac{19}{36}$
    $-\frac{6}{36}$

6. $\frac{9}{11}$
    $-\frac{2}{33}$

7. $\frac{10}{2}$
    $-\frac{4}{5}$

8. $\frac{90}{10}$
    $-\frac{12}{6}$

9. $\dfrac{36}{7}$
$-\dfrac{2}{3}$

11. $\dfrac{2}{4} - \dfrac{1}{4} =$

15. $\dfrac{14}{18} - \dfrac{6}{24} =$

19. $\dfrac{28}{7} - \dfrac{2}{3} =$

12. $\dfrac{8}{12} - \dfrac{3}{12} =$

16. $\dfrac{32}{8} - \dfrac{2}{4} =$

20. $\dfrac{14}{2} - \dfrac{4}{6} =$

10. $\dfrac{50}{10}$
$-\dfrac{30}{40}$

13. $\dfrac{4}{8} - \dfrac{3}{8} =$

17. $\dfrac{100}{50} - \dfrac{3}{5} =$

14. $\dfrac{5}{8} - \dfrac{1}{2} =$

18. $\dfrac{20}{15} - \dfrac{4}{5} =$

F. Multiply the following fractions. Convert answer to mixed numbers when possible and reduce fraction to lowest terms.

> **Rule:** 1. Convert mixed numbers to improper fractions.
> 2. Use cancellation and division to reduce the size of numbers in numerators or denominators.
> 3. Multiply numerators and denominators and reduce resulting fraction to lowest terms or convert to mixed number.

Examples:

$$\dfrac{1}{\cancel{6}_2} \times \dfrac{\cancel{3}^1}{5} = \dfrac{1}{10} \qquad 2\dfrac{3}{4} \times 4\dfrac{1}{2} = \dfrac{11}{4} \times \dfrac{9}{2} = \dfrac{99}{8} = 12\dfrac{3}{8}$$

Hints on Cancellation:

1. Look for powers of 10 (cross out zero(s))

Examples:

a. $\dfrac{\overset{7}{\overset{\cancel{35}}{\cancel{175,000}}}}{\underset{8}{\underset{\cancel{40}}{\cancel{200,000}}}} \times \dfrac{1}{}$ (Divide by 5) $= \dfrac{7}{8}$
(then by another 5)

OR

$\dfrac{\overset{7}{\cancel{175,000}}}{\underset{8}{\cancel{200,000}}} \times \dfrac{1}{}$ (Divide by 25) $= \dfrac{7}{8}$

b.
$$\overset{29\cancel{0}}{290} \times \frac{1}{\underset{1}{\cancel{1000}}} \times \frac{\overset{10}{\overset{1}{\cancel{500}}}}{\underset{1}{\cancel{50}}} \times \frac{6\cancel{0}}{1} = 29 \times 6 = 174 \quad \text{Cross out zeros}$$

OR

$$\overset{58}{\underset{2}{\cancel{290}}} \times \frac{1}{\cancel{1000}} \times \frac{\overset{1}{\cancel{500}}}{\underset{1}{\cancel{50}}} \times \frac{6\cancel{0}}{1} = 58 \times 6 = \frac{348}{2} = 174$$

2. Any even numbers—such as 58, 2, or 6—can always be divided by 2.

Example:

$$\overset{58}{\underset{2}{\underset{1}{\cancel{290}}}} \times \frac{1}{\cancel{1000}} \times \frac{\overset{1}{\cancel{500}}}{\underset{1}{\cancel{50}}} \times \frac{\overset{3}{\cancel{60}}}{1} = 58 \times 3 = 174 \quad \text{OR} \quad 29 \times 6 = 174$$

either divide the 2 into 6 or 2 into 58

3. If the sum of the digits in a number can be divided by a certain number, then that number divides into the original number.

Examples:

$$84 \times \frac{1}{2.2} \times \frac{8}{1} \times \frac{\overset{1}{\cancel{5}}}{\underset{15}{\cancel{75}}} \times \frac{5}{1}$$

If the sum of the digits in a number can be divided by 3, then 3 divides into the original number.

84 is 8 + 4 = 12
since 12 ÷ 3 is 4 (not a fraction)

$$\text{then} \quad 3\overline{\smash{)}84} \\ \underline{6} \\ 24 \\ \underline{24}$$
(quotient 28)

$$\overset{28}{\cancel{84}} \times \frac{1}{\cancel{2.2}} \times \frac{8}{1} \times \frac{\overset{1}{\cancel{5}}}{\underset{\underset{5}{\underset{1}{\cancel{15}}}}{\cancel{75}}} \times \frac{\overset{1}{\cancel{5}}}{1}$$

now divide 28 or 8 and 2.2 by 2 (Example shows 8 and 2.2 divided by 2)

$$\frac{\overset{28}{\cancel{84}}}{} \times \frac{1}{\underset{1.1}{\cancel{2.2}}} \times \frac{\overset{4}{\cancel{8}}}{1} \times \frac{\overset{1}{\cancel{5}}}{\underset{\underset{1}{\underset{\cancel{5}}{\cancel{15}}}}{\cancel{75}}} \times \frac{\overset{1}{\cancel{5}}}{1} = \frac{112}{1.1} = 1.1$$

$$\begin{array}{r} 10\ 1.818 \\ 1.1\overline{)112.0,000} \\ \underline{11} \\ 20 \\ \underline{11} \\ 90 \\ \underline{88} \\ 20 \\ \underline{11} \\ 90 \end{array}$$

$$\frac{112}{1.1} = 102$$

or 101.8

or 101.82

Practice:

1. $\dfrac{6}{7} \times \dfrac{3}{5} =$

2. $\dfrac{1}{4} \times \dfrac{3}{5} =$

3. $\dfrac{8}{10} \times \dfrac{1}{4} =$

4. $6\dfrac{2}{3} \times 5\dfrac{1}{2} =$

5. $5 \times 3\dfrac{2}{10} =$

6. $9 \times 3\dfrac{2}{3} =$

7. $6\dfrac{3}{7} \times 8 =$

8. $3\dfrac{2}{5} \times 20 =$

9. $4\dfrac{1}{6} \times 5\dfrac{1}{4} =$

10. $2\dfrac{6}{10} \times 1\dfrac{9}{10} =$

G. Divide the following fractions. Convert answer to mixed numbers when possible and reduce fraction to lowest terms.

> **Rule:** 1. Convert mixed numbers to improper fractions.
> 2. Invert the second fraction.
> 3. Cancel numerator and denominator wherever possible.
> 4. Multiply numerator and denominator and reduce resulting fraction to lowest terms or convert to mixed number.

Example:

$$\frac{1}{10} \div \frac{35}{5} = \frac{1}{\overset{}{\underset{2}{10}}} \times \frac{\overset{1}{\cancel{5}}}{3} = \frac{1}{6}$$

$$5\frac{3}{4} \div 3\frac{1}{6} = \frac{23}{\underset{2}{\cancel{4}}} \times \frac{\overset{3}{\cancel{6}}}{19} = \frac{69}{38} = 1\frac{31}{38}$$

Practice:

1. $\dfrac{1}{4} \div \dfrac{2}{16} =$

2. $\dfrac{1}{2} \div \dfrac{3}{2} =$

3. $\dfrac{3}{6} \div \dfrac{22}{23} =$

4. $\dfrac{32}{4} \div 2 =$

5. $6\dfrac{2}{4} \div 4 =$

6. $2\dfrac{2}{5} \div 1\dfrac{3}{15} =$

7. $4\dfrac{2}{4} \div 3\dfrac{1}{2} =$

8. $2\dfrac{2}{8} \div 3\dfrac{4}{8} =$

9. $4\dfrac{6}{18} \div \dfrac{4}{8} =$

10. $20\dfrac{1}{2} \div 6\dfrac{1}{6} =$

Note: When multiplying complex fractions, it is necessary to use both the multiplication and division rules for fractions.

Examples:

a. $\dfrac{1}{6} \times \dfrac{20}{1/4} \times \dfrac{1}{15}$

Take $\dfrac{20}{1/4}$ to the side and get a simpler fraction.

$\dfrac{20}{1/4}$ means 20 divided by 1/4 or $20 \div \dfrac{1}{4} = 20 \times \dfrac{4}{1} = 80$

So, $\dfrac{1}{6} \times \dfrac{20}{1/4} \times \dfrac{1}{15}$ becomes $\dfrac{1}{\underset{3}{\cancel{6}}} \times \overset{\overset{8}{\cancel{16}}}{\cancel{80}} \times \dfrac{1}{\underset{3}{\cancel{15}}} = \dfrac{8}{9}$ or 0.889 or 0.89 or 0.9

OR change $\dfrac{1}{4}$ to 0.25

$$\dfrac{1}{6} \times \dfrac{20}{1/4} \times \dfrac{1}{15} = \dfrac{1}{\cancel{6}^{\,3}} \times \dfrac{\cancel{20}^{\,\overset{2}{\cancel{4}}}}{.25} \times \dfrac{1}{\cancel{15}^{\,3}} = \dfrac{2}{2.25} =$$

$$\begin{array}{r} .88 \\ 2.25\overline{)2.00{.}00} \\ 180 \\ \hline 2000 \\ 1800 \\ \hline \end{array}$$

b. $\dfrac{1}{100} \times \dfrac{1}{1/150} \times \dfrac{15}{1}$

$\quad 1 \div \dfrac{1}{150} = 1 \times \dfrac{150}{1} = 150$

$\quad = \dfrac{1}{\cancel{100}_{\,2}} \times \dfrac{\cancel{150}^{\,3}}{1} \times \dfrac{15}{1} = \dfrac{45}{2} = 22.5$

OR change $\dfrac{1}{150}$ to a decimal as shown in previous example

$$\dfrac{1}{100} \times \dfrac{1}{1/150} \times \dfrac{15}{1}$$

$$\dfrac{1}{150} = \begin{array}{r} .0066 \\ 150\overline{)1.0000} \\ 900 \\ \hline 1000 \\ 900 \\ \hline \end{array}$$
   Because $\dfrac{1}{150}$ equals a repeating decimal, it is not a good idea to use this method here.

Note: To multiply fractions containing decimals in numerator or denominator, see the following examples.

Examples:

a. $0.2 \times \dfrac{1000}{1} \times \dfrac{1}{400}$

Divide 200 into 1000 and 400

$0.2 \times \dfrac{\overset{5}{\cancel{1000}}}{1} \times \dfrac{1}{\underset{2}{\cancel{400}}}$

either divide 2 into 0.2 (see section on dividing decimals)

$2\overline{).2}^{\;.1}$

$\overset{0.1}{0.\cancel{2}} \times \dfrac{\overset{5}{\cancel{1000}}}{1} \times \dfrac{1}{\underset{\underset{1}{\cancel{2}}}{\cancel{400}}} = 0.5$

OR

multiply 0.2×5 to 1.0 (see section on multiplying decimals)

$0.2 \times \dfrac{\overset{5}{\cancel{1000}}}{1} \times \dfrac{1}{\underset{2}{\cancel{400}}}$

$1.0 \times \dfrac{1}{2} = \dfrac{1}{2}$

b. $.006 \times \dfrac{\overset{15}{\cancel{60}}}{1} \times \dfrac{1}{\underset{.1}{\cancel{0.4}}}$ divide 4 into 60 and 0.4

$= \dfrac{.090}{0.1} = 0.9 \qquad \begin{array}{r} 15 \\ \times .006 \\ \hline .090 \end{array} \qquad \begin{array}{r} .90 \\ .1\overline{)0.90} \\ \underline{9} \end{array}$ or 0.9

c. $\overset{3}{\cancel{150}} \times \dfrac{1}{\underset{20}{\cancel{1000}}} \times \dfrac{1}{\underset{0.25}{\cancel{0.75}}} \times \dfrac{\overset{30}{\cancel{30}}}{1} = \dfrac{3}{.50} = 6 \qquad \begin{array}{r} 6 \\ .50\overline{)3.00} \\ \underline{300} \end{array}$

Decimals

A. Write the following decimals in numbers.

> **Rule:** Whole numbers are placed to the left of the decimal point; decimal fractions* are placed to the right of the decimal point.
>
> *A decimal fraction is defined by its location to the right of the decimal point (e.g., one place = tenths, two places = hundredths, three places = thousandths, four places = ten-thousandths).

Example: one and two tenths = 1.2
    three and five hundredths = 3.05

Note: The decimal point is read as *and*.

Practice:

1. twenty-four and 2 tenths
2. ten and 4 tenths
3. sixteen and twenty-nine hundredths
4. thirty and fifteen hundredths
5. two hundred sixty-one thousandths
6. three and three thousandths
7. nine ten-thousandths
8. thirty-two and twenty-seven ten-thousandths
9. six hundred-thousandths
10. twenty-five and eighty-five hundred-thousandths

B. Change the following decimals to fractions.

> **Rule:** 1. The numerator consists of the number(s) to the right of the decimal point.
> 2. The denominator consists of the decimal fraction (i.e., number of places to the right of the decimal point).
>
> **Example:**
>
> 1 = tenths (10), 2 = hundredths (100), etc.
>
> *Note:* The number of zeros in the denominator is always the same as the number of digits in the numerator.

Example: $0.1 = \dfrac{1}{10}$ $0.01 = \dfrac{1}{100}$

Practice:

1. 0.5	4. 0.25	7. 0.548	10. 0.7246
2. 0.4	5. 0.16	8. 0.973	
3. 0.53	6. 0.35	9. 0.4535	

C. Change the following fractions to decimals. Carry each answer to two decimal places and round to the nearest tenth.

Rule: Divide the numerator by the denominator.

Example: $\dfrac{5}{8} = 5 \div 8 = 8\overline{)5.000}$

$$\begin{array}{r} .625 \\ \hline 4\ 8 \\ \hline 20 \\ 16 \\ \hline 40 \\ 40 \\ \hline \end{array}$$

$\dfrac{5}{8}$ = 0.625 or 0.6 to nearest tenth

or 0.63 to nearest hundredth

Practice:

1. $\dfrac{1}{3}$ 6. $\dfrac{12}{14}$

2. $\dfrac{1}{6}$ 7. $\dfrac{8}{16}$

3. $\dfrac{2}{5}$ 8. $\dfrac{5}{12}$

4. $\dfrac{5}{6}$ 9. $\dfrac{1}{4}$

5. $\dfrac{3}{4}$ 10. $\dfrac{14}{35}$

D. Add the following decimals.

Rule: 1. Place decimals to be added in a column with decimal points one under the other.
2. Add the columns and place the decimal point directly under the line of decimal points.

Example: 0.4
            +8.95
            ‾‾‾‾‾
            9.35

Practice:

1.   0.2
    +1.76
    ‾‾‾‾‾

2.   .50
      22.80
    + 7.00
    ‾‾‾‾‾‾‾

3.   .30
      3.615
    +11.2
    ‾‾‾‾‾

4.   16.
       2.345
       0.750
    +12.000
    ‾‾‾‾‾‾‾

5.   13.2
       6.215
       7.20
    +185.6
    ‾‾‾‾‾‾

6.   9.276
      10.31
     146.200
    +   8.3
    ‾‾‾‾‾‾‾

7.   6.03
       28.1
        7.2106
    +48.1
    ‾‾‾‾‾‾

8.   2470.50316
          4.3922
         61.74
    +   .111
    ‾‾‾‾‾‾‾‾‾‾

9.   0.000396
        21.25976
         8.71
    + 6.31256
    ‾‾‾‾‾‾‾‾‾

10.   62.132
          7.9204
          9.1
        168.0074
    +   .2183
    ‾‾‾‾‾‾‾‾‾

E. Subtract the following decimals.

Rule: 1. Place the decimals to be subtracted in a column with decimal points one under the other.

2. Subtract the columns and place the decimal point directly under the line of decimal points.

Example: 0.300*
            −0.106
            ‾‾‾‾‾
            0.194

*Zeros may be added after the decimal point without changing the value.

Practice:

1.   28.25
    − 6.10
    ‾‾‾‾‾‾

2. 386.152
    −   4.06
    ‾‾‾‾‾‾‾

3.　5.6
　　−3.92

4.　92.0064
　　− 2.84

5.　201.6002
　　− 29.364

6.　0.921
　　−0.070352

7.　24.92
　　− 8.0286

8.　17
　　− 6.2813

9.　793
　　− 24.008

10.　693.4228
　　− 16.111

F. Round off the following decimals to the place indicated.

Rule: 1. Carry computation to one decimal place beyond the desired place.
2. If the final digit is 4 or less, leave prior digit the same.
3. If the final digit is 5 or more, increase the prior digit by 1.

Example: Round to the nearest tenth:
$$7.01 = 7$$
Round to the nearest hundredth.
$$10.106 = 10.11$$

Practice:
1. 2.32 to nearest tenth
2. 3.44 to nearest tenth
3. 32.66 to nearest tenth
4. 16.791 to nearest hundredth
5. 41.105 to nearest hundredth
6. 15.4038 to nearest hundredth
7. 3.2896 to nearest thousandth
8. 291.6345 to nearest thousandth
9. 782.5211 to nearest tenth
10. 2.6859 to nearest tenth

G. Multiply the following decimals.

Rule: 1. Multiply as whole numbers.
2. Count the total number of decimal places in the problem.
3. Starting from the right, count off the same number of places in the answer.
4. If necessary, add zeros to provide enough places in the answer.

Example:

$$\begin{array}{r} 3.9 \quad \text{(1 decimal place)} \\ \times\,\underline{0.005} \quad \text{(3 decimal places)} \\ 0.0195 \quad \text{(4 decimal places)} \end{array}$$

Practice:

1. $\begin{array}{r} 16.3 \\ \times\;\underline{0.8} \end{array}$

2. $\begin{array}{r} 32.6 \\ \times\underline{0.25} \end{array}$

3. $\begin{array}{r} 93.6 \\ \times\;\underline{3.2} \end{array}$

4. $\begin{array}{r} 17.81 \\ \times\;\underline{6.02} \end{array}$

5. $\begin{array}{r} 71.3 \\ \times\underline{84.2} \end{array}$

6. $\begin{array}{r} 0.025 \\ \times\;\underline{0.2} \end{array}$

7. $\begin{array}{r} 0.087 \\ \times\;\underline{0.6} \end{array}$

8. $\begin{array}{r} 0.09302 \\ \times\;\underline{2.4} \end{array}$

9. $\begin{array}{r} 0.234 \\ \times\;\underline{7} \end{array}$

10. $\begin{array}{r} 2.361 \\ \times\;\underline{9} \end{array}$

H. Divide the following decimals. Carry to two decimal places and round to the nearest tenth.

Rule: 1. If the divisor is a whole number, proceed as in division of whole numbers. In the answer, place the decimal point directly above its position in the dividend.
2. If the divisor is a decimal, move the decimal point to the right end, making the divisor a whole number. Move the decimal point in the dividend the same number of places to the right (adding zeros if necessary). Then proceed as in division of whole numbers.

Example:

$$
\begin{array}{r}
3\ 33.33 \\
0.24\overline{\smash{)}80.00.00} \\
72\ \ \ \ \ \ \ \\
\overline{80\ \ \ \ \ } \\
72\ \ \ \ \ \\
\overline{80\ \ \ } \\
72\ \ \ \\
\overline{80\ } \\
72\ \\
\overline{80} \\
72 \\
\overline{8}
\end{array}
$$

Practice:

1. $2.5\overline{\smash{)}100.0}$

2. $3.24\overline{\smash{)}9.1006}$

3. $0.6\overline{\smash{)}1.75}$

4. $2.0\overline{\smash{)}9.0}$

5. $7.3\overline{\smash{)}62.59}$

6. $0.423 \div 3 =$

7. $1.5 \div 0.5 =$

8. $326.5 \div 22 =$

9. $222 \div 0.11 =$

10. $1.843 \div 20 =$

(*Note:* See Appendix C for answer key.)

Percentage Solutions

··

Objectives

Upon completion of this optional unit of study you should be able to:
- *Identify equivalent units for solids and liquids.*
- *Apply the label factor method to calculation of the precise amounts of solvent and/or solute necessary to prepare a solution of specified percentage strength.*

A solution is a liquid preparation containing one or more dissolved or diluted substances. The diluting fluid is called the *solvent* and the drug or other substance being dissolved is called the *solute*.

To prepare a specified percentage strength of a solution, it is necessary to calculate the exact amount of drug that must be added to a certain volume of liquid to produce a solution of the desired strength.

As a rule, percentage solutions are prepared by the pharmacist if they are not commercially available. Occasionally, it may be necessary for the nurse to prepare a percentage solution to be used for patient care or for disinfection (e.g., mouth rinse, throat irrigation, wet dressing, enema, douche) or for terminal disinfection of hospital equipment and contaminated areas. The label factor method can be used to calculate the amounts of solvent and solute necessary to prepare these solutions.

Equivalent Units for Solids and Liquids

In solutions, the word percent or the symbol % means the *parts of substance per 100 parts of solution*. For example, 2% indicates two parts of 100 parts total. The measured parts either must be units of the *same kind* or else must be *equivalents*. Certainly 2 grams of salt in 100 pounds of mixture could not be called a 2% mixture as grams and pounds are not equivalent units. The parts can be minims, drams, fluid ounces, cups, milliliters, or liters, for instance. For example, a 10% solution of alcohol means 10 parts of alcohol to 100 parts of solution. Because they are both liquids, the parts that measure both the alcohol and the total solution would be of the same kind. For instance, the solution could have 10 minims of alcohol for 100 minims of solution, 10 fluid ounces of alcohol for 100 fluid ounces of solution, or 10 pints of alcohol for 100 pints of solution. However, if a dry substance were to be placed into solution, equivalent units relating dry measure to liquid measure must be used. For example, a 5% salt solution would require 5 grains of salt for 100 minims of solution, 5 grams of salt for 100 milliliters of solution, or 5 ounces of salt for 100 fluid ounces of solution. It is important in this case to know the equivalents for dry and liquid measure, which are listed below.

EQUIVALENTS

DRY UNITS	FLUID UNITS
grain	minim
gram	milliliter
dram	fluid dram
ounce	fluid ounce
kilogram	liter

Calculation of Percentage Solutions Using Label Factor Method

The percentage strength of a desired solution is expressed as a conversion factor that contains the relationship between solute and solvent.

Examples:

a. Find the quantity of alcohol needed to prepare 200 ml of a 15% alcohol solution. The parts (solute and solvent) will be measured in ml. The conversion factor can be written as:

$$\frac{15 \text{ ml alcohol}}{100 \text{ ml solution}} \text{ or } \frac{100 \text{ ml solution}}{15 \text{ ml alcohol}}$$

Problem: the quantity of alcohol needed to prepare 200 ml of solution.

Definite quantity: 200 ml of solution. This is the starting factor and the problem proceeds as follows:

Starting Factor   Answer Label
200 ml solution   ml alcohol
Equivalent: 15 ml alcohol = 100 ml solution

Conversion Equation:

$$200 \text{ ml solution} \times \frac{15 \text{ ml alcohol}}{100 \text{ ml solution}} = 30 \text{ ml alcohol}$$

(*Note:* In this problem, not only are the units labeled as ml but also the substances are clearly identified.) **Remember: It is extremely im-**

portant that the quantity of total solution is not confused with the quantity of substance dissolved; therefore, the descriptive label should be used.

b. Find the quantity of 25% solution needed to supply 15 grains of drug.
   Starting Factor   Answer Label
      15 gr drug   m solution
   Equivalent: 25 gr drug = 100 m solution

Conversion Equation: $15 \, \cancel{\text{gr drug}} \times \dfrac{100 \text{ m solution}}{25 \, \cancel{\text{gr drug}}} = 60 \text{ m solution}$

(*Note:* In the second factor, grains of drug has to appear in the denominator to *cancel the label* of the first factor. However, the relationship 100 minims of solution to 25 grains of drug is an equivalent expression and gives a true relationship even when inverted.)

c. Find the number of grams of dry drug needed to prepare 60 ml of 5% solution.
   Starting Factor   Answer Label
   60 ml solution   Gm drug
   Equivalent: 5 Gm drug = 100 ml solution

Conversion Equation: $60 \, \cancel{\text{ml solution}} \times \dfrac{5 \text{ Gm drug}}{100 \, \cancel{\text{ml solution}}} = 3 \text{ Gm}$

d. Find the volume of 10% solution that can be made using four 5-grain tablets of drug.
   Starting Factor   Answer Label
      4 tablets   m solution
   Equivalents: 5 gr drug = 1 tab, 10 gr drug = 100 m solution

Conversion Equation:

$4 \, \cancel{\text{tabs}} \times \dfrac{5 \, \cancel{\text{gr drug}}}{1 \, \cancel{\text{tab}}} \times \dfrac{100 \text{ m solution}}{10 \, \cancel{\text{gr drug}}} = 200 \text{ m solution}$

e. Find the number of 10 grain tablets needed to make a pint of 2% solution of drug.
   Starting Factor   Answer Label
      1 pt solution   tablets
   Equivalents: 1 pt = 1 oz, 2 oz drug = 100 oz solution, 1 oz = 8 ℨ,
              1 ℨ = 60 gr, 10 gr = 1 tab

Conversion Equation:

$$1 \, \text{pt solution} \times \frac{16 \, \text{oz}}{1 \, \text{pt}} \times \frac{2 \, \text{oz drug}}{100 \, \text{oz solution}} \times \frac{8 \, \text{dr}}{1 \, \text{oz}} \times \frac{60 \, \text{gr}}{1 \, \text{dr}} \times \frac{1 \, \text{tab}}{10 \, \text{gr}} = 15.3$$

or 15 tablets

f. Prepare 2500 ml of a 1:1000 solution using 1 Gm tablets.

Starting Factor   Answer Label
    2500 ml   tablets
Equivalents: 1 Gm = 1000 ml, 1 Gm = 1 tab

Conversion Equation:

$$2500 \, \text{ml solution} \times \frac{1 \, \text{Gm drug}}{1000 \, \text{ml solution}} \times \frac{1 \, \text{tab}}{1 \, \text{Gm drug}} = 2.5 \text{ tablets}$$

(*Note:* Solution strength may be expressed either as percentage or as a ratio. The ratio 1:1000 means there is one part solute in 1000 parts of solvent and the conversion factor in the above problem is written as $\frac{1 \, \text{Gm drug}}{1000 \, \text{ml solution}}$.)

Self-Quiz—Equivalents

Match dry units with equivalent fluid units.

_____ 1. grain   A. fluid dram

_____ 2. gram   B. fluid ounce

_____ 3. dram   C. liter

_____ 4. ounce   D. milliliter

_____ 5. kilogram   E. minim

Practice: Calculation of Percentage Solutions

1. How many ml of solute are needed to prepare 4000 ml of a 2% Lysol solution?

2. How many grams of solute are needed to prepare 2 oz of 8% iodine solution?

3. Prepare 1000 ml of 70% alcohol solution.

4. Prepare 1000 ml of 1% Neomycin solution from 5 Gm Neomycin tablets.

5. Prepare 4000 ml 1:1000 bichloride of mercury solution using 500 mg tablets.

6. Prepare 500 ml 1:2000 potassium permanganate solution using potassium permanganate crystals (measure in Gm).

7. Prepare 1000 ml 1:100 potassium permanganate solution using potassium permanganate crystals (measure in Gm).

8. Prepare 250 ml 1% acetic acid solution from a 10% solution.

9. Prepare 2000 ml of 1 : 1000 bichloride of mercury solution using 0.5 Gm tablets.

10. How many ml of alcohol are needed to prepare 1 qt of 40% alcohol solution?

Answer Key

Self-Quiz—Equivalents (page 346)
1. E
2. D
3. A
4. B
5. C

Practice: Calculation of Percentage Solutions (pages 346–348)
1. 80 ml Lysol/3920 ml water
2. 4.8 Gm iodine
3. 700 ml alcohol/300 ml water
4. 2 Neomycin tab/1000 ml water
5. 8 bichloride of mercury tab/4000 ml water
6. 0.25 Gm potassium permanganate crystals/500 ml water
7. 10 Gm potassium permanganate crystals/1000 ml water
8. 25 ml acetic acid/225 ml water
9. 4 bichloride of mercury tab/2000 ml water
10. 400 ml alcohol/600 ml water

Answer Keys

....

Unit 1   The Label Factor Method

Practice: Identifying the Starting Factor and Answer Label (page 5)

	STARTING FACTOR	ANSWER LABEL
1.	3 gr	mg
2.	5 kg	lb
3.	250 mg	tab
4.	0.5 Gm	cap
5.	250 mg	ml

Practice: Setting Up Conversion Equations (pages 12–13)

1. Equivalents: 500 mg = 1 tsp, 1 tsp = 5 ml

   Conversion Equation: $250 \;\cancel{mg} \times \dfrac{1 \;\cancel{tsp}}{500 \;\cancel{mg}} \times \dfrac{5 \;ml}{1 \;\cancel{tsp}} =$ _____ ml

2. Equivalents: 250 mg = 5 ml, 1 ml = 15 m

   Conversion Equation: $125 \;\cancel{mg} \times \dfrac{5 \;\cancel{ml}}{250 \;\cancel{mg}} \times \dfrac{15 \;m}{1 \;\cancel{ml}} =$ _____ m

3. Equivalents: 0.5 Gm = ʒ 1, ʒ 1 = 4 ml

   Conversion Equation: $0.75 \;\cancel{Gm} \times \dfrac{ʒ 1}{0.5 \;\cancel{Gm}} \times \dfrac{4 \;ml}{ʒ 1} =$ _____ ml

4. Equivalents: gr 1 = 60 mg, 1 tab = 15 mg

   Conversion Equation: $\cancel{gr} \;1/8 \times \dfrac{60 \;\cancel{mg}}{\cancel{gr}\,1} \times \dfrac{1 \;tab}{15 \;\cancel{mg}} =$ _____ tab

5. Equivalents: 5 ml = 1 tsp, 1 tsp = 300 mg

   Conversion Equation: $15 \;\cancel{ml} \times \dfrac{1 \;\cancel{tsp}}{5 \;\cancel{ml}} \times \dfrac{300 \;mg}{1 \;\cancel{tsp}} =$ _____ mg

Practice: *Solving Conversion Equations (pages 14–15)*

1. Equivalents: 0.125 mg = 1 tab

   Conversion Equation: $0.250 \text{ mg} \times \dfrac{1 \text{ tab}}{0.125 \text{ mg}} = 2 \text{ tab}$

2. Equivalents: 30 mg = 1 cap, 60 mg = gr 1

   Conversion Equation: $\text{gr } \frac{1}{2} \times \dfrac{60 \text{ mg}}{\text{gr } 1} \times \dfrac{1 \text{ cap}}{30 \text{ mg}} = 1 \text{ cap}$

3. Equivalents: 0.5 Gm = 1 tab, 1000 mg = 1 Gm

   Conversion Equation: $250 \text{ mg} \times \dfrac{1 \text{ Gm}}{1000 \text{ mg}} \times \dfrac{1 \text{ tab}}{0.5 \text{ Gm}} = 0.5 \text{ tab}$

4. Equivalents: gr ¼ = 20 m, 15 m = 1 ml

   Conversion Equation: $\text{gr } \frac{1}{6} \times \dfrac{20 \text{ m}}{\text{gr } \frac{1}{4}} \times \dfrac{1 \text{ ml}}{15 \text{ m}} = 0.89 \text{ ml}$

5. Equivalents: gr ¹⁄₁₅₀ = 1 ml, 1 ml = 15 m

   Conversion Equation: $\text{gr } \frac{1}{100} \times \dfrac{1 \text{ ml}}{\text{gr } \frac{1}{150}} \times \dfrac{15 \text{ m}}{1 \text{ ml}} = 22.5 \text{ m}$

   OR

   $\text{gr } 0.01 \times \dfrac{1 \text{ ml}}{\text{gr } 0.007} \times \dfrac{15 \text{ m}}{1 \text{ ml}} = 21 \text{ m}$

6. Equivalents: gr 7.5 = 5 ml, 15 gr = 1 Gm

   Conversion Equation: $1 \text{ Gm} \times \dfrac{15 \text{ gr}}{1 \text{ Gm}} \times \dfrac{5 \text{ ml}}{\text{gr } 7.5} = 10 \text{ ml}$

7. Equivalents: 400 mg = 1 tsp, 5 ml = 1 tsp

   Conversion Equation: $10 \text{ ml} \times \dfrac{1 \text{ tsp}}{5 \text{ ml}} \times \dfrac{400 \text{ mg}}{1 \text{ tsp}} = 800 \text{ mg}$

8. Equivalents: 125 mg = 5 ml

   Conversion Equation: $200 \text{ mg} \times \dfrac{5 \text{ ml}}{125 \text{ mg}} = 8 \text{ ml}$

9. Equivalents: 30 mg = 5 ml

   Conversion Equation: $75 \text{ mg} \times \dfrac{5 \text{ ml}}{30 \text{ mg}} = 12.5 \text{ ml}$

10. Equivalents: gr 1 ½ = 1 tab, gr 1 = 60 mg

   Conversion Equation: $90 \text{ mg} \times \dfrac{\text{gr} 1}{60 \text{ mg}} \times \dfrac{1 \text{ tab}}{\text{gr} 1.5} = 1 \text{ tab}$

Unit 2   The Metric System of Measurement

Practice: Convert Within the Metric System (pages 21–23)
1. 3.2 L
2. 0.4 Gm
3. 2 kg
4. 5 mg
5. 0.3 M
6. 750 ml
7. 220 mg
8. 2500 Gm
9. 2.5 cm
10. 12,000 mcg

Unit 3   The Apothecaries System of Measurement

Practice: Abbreviations (page 26)
1. ℥
2. gr
3. m
4. s̄s̄
5. ʒ

Practice: Convert Within the Apothecaries System (pages 28–29)
1. 1 ⁷⁄₁₀ qt
2. ½ oz or ℥ s̄s̄
3. 24 oz or ℥ 24
4. ½ dr or ʒ s̄s̄
5. ½ dr or ʒ s̄s̄
6. 10 dr or ʒ x
7. ³⁄₁₀ oz or ℥ ³⁄₁₀
8. 256 dr or ʒ 256
9. 56 oz or ℥ 56
10. 3 ⁹⁄₁₀ lb

Unit 4   The Household System of Measurement

Practice: Abbreviations (page 31)
1. gtt
2. gal
3. pt
4. tbsp
5. tsp

Practice: Convert Within the Household System (pages 33–34)

1. 48 tsp
2. 256 oz
3. 16 cups
4. 5.7 ft
5. 2 oz
6. 18 tsp
7. 2.8 gal
8. 41.6 oz
9. 8.3 oz
10. 12 tbsp

Unit 5   Conversion of Metric, Apothecaries, and Household Units

Self-Quiz—Equivalents

A. Fill in the Blanks (pages 35–36)

1. 1 gr
2. 1 Gm
3. 1000 mg
4. 1000 Gm
5. 2.2 lb
6. 1 gtt
7. 1000 ml
8. 2.5 cm
9. 39.4 in
10. ½ oz

B. Match Equivalent Amounts (page 36)

1. d
2. c
3. e
4. b
5. a

Practice (pages 39–44)

1. 1250 ml
2. 88 lb
3. 2.5 cups
4. 10 ml
5. 30 mg
6. 1.4 kg
7. 1.3 ml
8. 8 tbsp
9. ʒ 19.2
10. 30 gr
11. 90 gtt
12. 75 m
13. 2 gr
14. 0.7 ml
15. 2.5 tsp
16. 22.5 ml
17. 480 ml
18. ʒ 7.5
19. 8 Gm
20. 71.4 kg
21. 180 mg
22. 45 m
23. 11.4 lb
24. 12 cm
25. 24 in
26. ʒ 64
27. 1.5 gr
28. 82.5 gr
29. 4 tbsp
30. 300 mg

Unit 6   Calculation of Oral Medications

Practice: Reading Labels (pages 51–54)

A. Figure 6-6

1. Inderal LA 80
2. Propranolol Hydrochloride
3. 80 mg/cap

4. capsule
5. Ayerst

6. 1
7. 2

B. Figure 6-7

1. None
2. Potassium Chloride
3. 15 mEq/11.25 ml
4. liquid
5. Roxane

6. 11.25
7. 7.5 ml

C. Figure 6-8

1. None
2. Nitroglycerin
3. 0.6 mg (gr 1/100)/tab
4. tablet
5. Lilly

D. Figure 6-9

1. Nitro-Bid
2. Nitroglycerin
3. 2.5 mg/cap
4. capsule
5. Marion

	NITROGLYCERIN TABLETS	**NITRO-BID PLATEAU CAPS**
Route	sublingual	oral
Dosage Strength	0.6 mg or gr 1/100	2.5 mg
Form	tablet	capsule
Manufacturer	Lilly	Marion

Practice: Reading Labels and Clinical Calculations Involving Medications Administered by the Oral Route (po) (pages 54–57)

1. 2 tab
2. 1 cap
3. 12 ml
4. nystatin, 500,000 U
5. prochlorperazine maleate, 2 tab

Practice: Oral Dosage Based on Body Weight (pages 59–60)
1. 2 tab
2. 3 cap
3. 14.6 ml
4. 4.5 tab
5. 2 tab

Practice: Clinical Calculations Involving Medications Administered by the Oral Route (po) (pages 60–70)

1. 3 tab	11. 14.1 ml	21. 3 tab	31. 1 tab	41. 1 tab
2. 6 ml	12. 3 tab	22. 2.5 ml	32. 2 cap	42. 3 tab
3. 2 tab	13. 3 tab	23. 1 cap	33. 2 tab	43. 0.5 tab
4. 2.4 ml	14. 2 cap	24. 8 ml	34. 4 ml	44. 20 ml
5. 2 tab	15. 6.8 ml	25. 4 tab	35. 3 tsp	45. 20 ml
6. 0.5 tab	16. 10 ml	26. 0.5 tab	36. 2.5 ml	46. 12.5 ml
7. 0.5 tab	17. 3 tab	27. 1.5 tab	37. 8 ml	47. 4 tab
8. 4 cap	18. 0.5 tab	28. 2.5 ml	38. 1.2 ml	48. 1 tab
9. 2 dr	19. 0.25 tab	29. 0.5 tab	39. 2 tab	49. 2 tab
10. 15 ml	20. 2 cap	30. 1 tab	40. 2 cap	50. 2 tab

Unit 7 Administration of Oral Medications

Self-Quiz—Abbreviations (pages 75-76)
A. Match the abbreviations with correct meaning

1. c	6. l
2. b	7. f
3. i	8. n
4. e	9. h
5. a	10. d

B. Write the Term

1. before meals	6. without
2. capsule	7. elixir
3. gram	8. whenever necessary
4. after meals	9. one-half
5. every three hours	10. milliliter

C. Identify the Route

1. intramuscular	6. both eyes
2. intravenous	7. by mouth
3. subcutaneous	8. sublingual
4. left eye	9. intradermal
5. right eye	

Practice: Simulated Medication Administration Using Medex (pages 85–89)

1.

MEDICATION	AMOUNT TO BE GIVEN
Digoxin	0.25 mg
K-Lor	20 mEq
Alupent Syrup	1.5 tsp
Erythromycin D-R	500 mg
Haldol	1.5 mg or 0.75 ml

2. 2 tab at 7:30 A.M.
3. ■ water or juice
   ■ 120 ml
4. ■ 12.5 mg/tab
   ■ 2 tab
5. ■ 7.5 ml
   ■ 15 mg
   ■ yes
6. ■ 15 ml
   ■ 20 doses

7. ■ 100 mg/cap
   ■ 1 cap
8. ■ 4 mg
   ■ 2 mg
9. ■ Darvocet-N 100
   ■ every 4 hours as needed
   ■ 1 tab
   ■ July 1, 1993

Unit 8   Calculation of Parenteral Medications

Shade in the Dosage (page 94)

Reading of 3 Syringes

No. 1

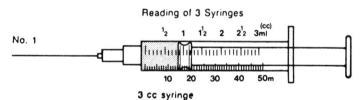

3 cc syringe

No. 2

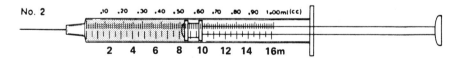

Tuberculin

No. 3

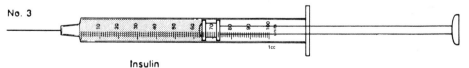

Insulin

Practice: Reading Labels (pages 101–103)

1. (Ticarcillin DiSodium)
   a. 3 Gm
   b. 6 ml
   c. 2.6 ml = 1 Gm
2. (Geopen)
   a. IV or IM
   b. 20 ml
   c. 2.5 ml
3. (20 million units)
   a. IV only
   b. refrigerator
   c. 9/23
4. (1 Gm every 4–6 hours)
   a. 5.7 ml
   b. 2 ml
   c. 24 hours
5. (IM)
   a. 100 mg
   b. IM
   c. Vistaril

6. (2–12 Gm daily)
   a. 5 ml
   b. sterile water for injection
   c. IV, IM, IP
7. (Nembutal)
   a. single
   b. gr 1½
   c. 100 mg
8. (10 ml)
   a. 50 mg/cc
   b. Oxytetracycline
   c. Roerig
9. (Thiothixene Hydrochloride)
   a. IM
   b. no
   c. 2 ml

Practice: Calculating Dosages from Pre-Mixed Solutions (pages 107–115)

1. 0.6 ml
2. 1.5 ml, hydroxyzine hydrochloride
3. 1.5 ml or 1.7 ml
4. 0.5 ml, glycopyrrolate
5. 1.5 ml, penicillin G procaine
6. 0.6 ml, ampicillin sodium
7. 0.5 ml, kanamycin sulfate
8. 0.7 ml, dimenhydrinate
9. 0.5 ml, Lanoxin
10. 0.5 ml

11. 1.6 ml
12. 1.6 ml
13. 0.8 ml
14. 2 ml
15. 1 ml
16. 3 ml
17. 0.8 ml
18. 0.8 ml
19. 1.5 ml
20. 1 ml

Practice: IM Calculations Based on Body Weight (pages 116–118)

1. 1.9 ml
2. 3.3 ml
3. 1.2 ml
4. 2.2 ml
5. 2 ml

6. 1.4 ml
7. 2.5 ml
8. 0.8 ml
9. 1.2 ml
10. 1.5 ml

Practice: Medications Dispensed in Units (pages 119–122)

1. 0.4 ml
2. 0.7 ml
3. 0.8 ml
4. 0.75 ml
5. 1.7 ml

6. 1.7 ml
7. 1.1 ml
8. 0.1 ml
9. 0.3 ml
10. 2.5 ml

Practice: Reconstitution of Drugs in Powder Form (pages 125–131)

1. ampicillin
   a. 3.5 ml
   b. read circular
   c. 250 mg/ml
   d. within 1 hr
   e. 1.4 ml
   f. 250–500 mg q 6 h
2. oxacillin
   a. sterile water for injection
   b. 5.7 ml
   c. 250 mg = 1.5 ml
   d. 1.8 ml
   e. 250–500 mg q 4–6 h
   f. ■ 10 A.M. on 9/19
      ■ 10 A.M. on 9/23
3. carbenicillin sodium
   a. sterile water for injection
   b. 1 Gm/2.5 ml
   c. ■ within 24 hr
      ■ within 72 hr
   d. 1.25 ml
   e. read circular
4. cephalothin sodium
   a. sterile water for injection
   b. 4 ml
   c. 0.5 Gm/2.2 ml
   d. 2.2 ml

   e. 2 Gm
   f. 2–12 Gm daily
   g. 9 A.M. on 11/13
   h. within 12 h
5. a. 4 ml
   b. 2 ml
   c. 1.6 ml
   d. 7 days in refrigerator
   e. refrigerator
   f. 300,000–600,000 U q 4h
   g. same
6. 0.6 ml
7. 2 ml
8. 2.2 ml
9. 2.5 ml
10. 2 ml
11. 1 ml
12. 1.6 ml
13. 2 ml
14. 3 ml
15. 2.5 ml
16. 4.4 ml
17. 1.5 ml
18. 0.9 ml
19. 2.1 ml
20. 1.6 ml

Unit 9   Administration of Parenteral Medications

Practice: Reading Insulin Labels (pages 153–156)

1. U 100
2. Lilly, Squibb-Novo

3. ■ a, d, g, h
   ■ g, h, i, k
   ■ p, q
   ■ b
   ■ c
   ■ f, o, p
4. ■ R
   ■ S
   ■ N
   ■ L
   ■ U
   ■ P

5. a. 1. a
      2. 24 U
   b. 1. j
      2. 45 U
   c. 1. b, q
      2. Regular (e)
      3. 48 U
   d. 1. c, j
      2. Lente (j)
      3. 66 U

Unit 10   Calculation of Intravenous Medications and Solutions

Reading Labels: Drop Factor (page 166)

A. Figure 10-4

1. a. 10
   b. 15
   c. 60

2. a, b
3. c

Reading IV Labels (pages 168–170)

A. Figure 10-5

1. 500 ml
2. 5%
3. Abbott

B. Figure 10-6

1. 250 ml
2. 0.9%

C. Figure 10-7

1. 1000 ml
2. 5%
3. NaCl, NaLactate, KCl, CaCl

Practice: Calculation of IV Flow Rate When Total Infusion Time Is Specified (pages 178–180)

1. 31 gtt
2. 25 gtt
3. 50 gtt
4. 23 gtt
5. 35 gtt

6. 52 gtt
7. 28 gtt
8. 6 gtt
9. 100 gtt
10. 13 gtt

Practice: Calculation of IV Flow Rate When Infusion Rate Is Specified (pages 180–182)

11. 31 gtt
12. 17 gtt
13. 38 gtt
14. 21 gtt

15. 125 gtt
16. 20 gtt
17. 13 gtt

Practice: Calculation of Flow Rate When IV Contains Medication (pages 182–183)

1. 63 gtt
2. 125 gtt
3. 25 gtt

4. 50 gtt
5. 33 gtt

Practice: Calculation of the Number of ML/HR That Will Infuse (pages 184–186)

1. 125 ml
2. 83 ml
3. 125 ml
4. 125 ml

5. 104 ml
6. 83 ml
7. 125 ml

Practice: Calculation of Infusion Time (pages 186–187)

1. 12 hr 30 min
2. 8 hr 54 min
3. 4 hr

4. 14 hr 42 min
5. 7 hr 12 min

Practice: Adding Drugs to IVs and Calculating Flow Rate in gtt/min (pages 190–196)

1. cefazolin sodium
   a. 2 ml
   b. 1.6 ml
   c. 25 gtt
2. a. 2.4 ml
   b. 125 gtt
3. Omnipen-N
   a. 3 ml
   b. 38 gtt
4. a. 15 ml
   b. 28 gtt
5. a. 3 ml
   b. 150 gtt

6. 121 gtt
7. a. 1 ml
   b. 17 gtt
8. a. 1.3 ml
   b. 25 gtt
9. a. 3.1 ml
   b. 167 gtt
10. a. 10 ml
    b. 28 gtt

Practice: Calculation of the Volume of Solution or Concentration of Drug (pages 198–204)

1. a. 2.5 ml
   b. 100 ml
2. 25 ml
3. 8 ml
4. 50 ml
5. 100 ml
6. 100 ml
7. 121 ml
8. a. 6 ml
   b. 71 ml

9. a. 300 ml
   b. 10 min
10. 50 mg
11. 4 mg
12. 3 mcg
13. 1.25 mEq
14. 96 mg
15. a. 10 ml
    b. 267 ml
    c. 2 hr 54 min

16. a. 40 ml
    b. 0.13 Gm
    c. 400 ml
    d. 8 hr
17. a. 15 ml
    b. 0.3 mg
    c. 20 ml
    d. 30 ml
    e. 40 ml

Practice: IV Flow Rate and Dosages Based on Body Weight (pages 206–210)

1. a. 459.1 mcg/min
   b. 55 ml/hr
   c. 55 gtt/min
   d. 8.3 mcg/gtt
2. a. 515.2 mcg/min
   b. 31 ml/hr
   c. 31 gtt/min
   d. 16.6 mcg/gtt

3. a. 135 mcg/min
   b. 41 ml/hr
   c. 41 gtt/min
   d. 3.3 mcg/gtt
4. a. 582.4 mcg/min
   b. 11 ml/hr
   c. 11 gtt/min
   d. 52.9 mcg/gtt

5. a. 416 mcg/min
   b. 15 ml/hr
   c. 15 gtt/min
   d. 27.7 mcg/gtt

Practice: Titration Infusions (pages 213–219)

1. a. 10,000 mcg/ml
   b. Lower: 3181.8 mcg/min
      Upper: 6363.6 mcg/min
   c. Lower: 19 ml/hr or
      19 gtt/min
      Upper: 38 ml/hr or
      38 gtt/min
   d. 167.5 mcg/gtt
   e. 4020 mcg/min
2. a. 800 mcg/ml
   b. Lower: 397.7 mcg/min
      Upper: 795.5 mcg/min
   c. Lower: 30 ml/hr or
      30 gtt/min
      Upper: 60 ml/hr or
      60 gtt/min
   d. 13.3 mcg/gtt
   e. 532 mcg/min

3. a. 5000 mcg/ml
   b. Lower: 350 mcg/min
      Upper: 700 mcg/min
   c. Lower: 4 ml/hr or
      4 gtt/min
      Upper: 8 ml/hr or
      8 gtt/min
   d. 87.5 mcg/gtt
   e. 787.5 mcg/min
4. a. 100 mcg/ml
   b. Lower: 136 mcg/min
      Upper: 272.7 mcg/min
   c. Lower: 82 ml/hr or
      82 gtt/min
      Upper: 164 ml/hr or
      164 gtt/min
   d. 1.7 mcg/gtt
   e. 130.9 mcg/min

5. a. 400 mcg/ml
    b. Lower: 150 mcg/min
        Upper: 375 mcg/min
    c. Lower: 23 ml/hr or
        23 gtt/min
        Upper: 56 ml/hr or
        56 gtt/min
    d. 6.5 mcg/gtt
    e. 182 mcg/min

Practice: IV Bolus (pages 220–224)

1. a. 0.8 ml
    b. 24 sec
2. a. 9.6 ml
    b. 9 min 36 sec
3. a. 2 ml
    b. 2 min
4. a. 0.6 ml
    b. 1 min 12 sec
5. a. 3.5 ml
    b. 1 min 48 sec

6. a. 306.8 mg
    b. 0.61 ml
    c. 12 min 18 sec
7. a. 77.3 mg
    b. 7.7 ml
    c. 2 min 12 sec
    d. 5 ml
    e. 30 ml

Practice: Nutrition Calculations (pages 226–228)

1. 255 kcal
2. 140 kcal
3. 110 kcal
4. 42.5 kcal
5. 420 kcal
6. 850 kcal

7. 600 kcal
8. 2040 kcal
9. a. 200 kcal
    b. 425 kcal
10. a. 170 kcal
    b. 340 kcal

Practice: Adjusting IVs (pages 230–234)

1. a. 35 gtt
    b. 33 gtt
2. a. 42 gtt
    b. 44 gtt
3. a. 42 gtt
    b. 33 gtt
4. a. 21 gtt
    b. 27 gtt
5. a. 63 gtt
    b. 50 gtt

6. a. 31 gtt
    b. 33 gtt
7. a. 28 gtt
    b. 32 gtt
8. a. 50 gtt
    b. 40 gtt
9. a. 35 gtt
    b. 31 gtt
10. a. 63 gtt
    b. 60 gtt

Unit 12   Pediatric Dosage

Practice: Calculating Pediatric Dosage Based on Body Weight—Oral Medications (pages 249–253)

1. digoxin, 7.6 ml
2. 5.3 ml
3. 6.8 ml
4. 5.5 ml
5. 7.5 ml
6. 5 ml
7. 9.3 ml
8. 9.5 ml
9. 4.5 ml
10. 5.1 ml
11. 13.2 ml
12. 1.7 ml
13. 6.4 ml
14. 0.6 ml
15. 2.1 ml
16. 1 ml

Practice: Calculating Pediatric Dosage—Injections (pages 254–257)

1. Kantrex, 1 ml
2. furosemide, 3.4 ml
3. 0.75 ml
4. 0.27 ml
5. 2.5 ml
6. 0.12 ml
7. 0.59 ml
8. 1.1 ml
9. 2.3 ml
10. 0.045 ml or 0.05 ml

Practice: Calculating Pediatric Dosage–IVs (pages 258–262)

1. a. 7.5 ml
   b. 978 mcg
   c. 58.7 mg
   d. 49 ml
   e. 5 hr 6 min
2. a. 1.2 ml
   b. 37 mcg
   c. 2.2 mg
   d. 18 ml/hr or
      19 ml/hr
3. a. 6.1 mg
   b. 0.24 ml
4. 0.36 ml
5. 3.3 ml
6. a. 12.1 ml
   b. 212 gtt
7. a. 0.76 ml
   b. 300 gtt
8. a. 0.87 ml
   b. 200 gtt

Practice: Use the Nomogram to Determine Child's BSA (page 264)

1. 1.22 M^2
2. 0.8 M^2
3. 1.1 M^2
4. 0.47 M^2
5. 0.53 M^2

Practice: Use Nomogram and Label Factor Method to Calculate Pediatric Dosages (pages 265–266)

1. 10.3 mg
2. 4.4 mg
3. 101.2 mg
4. 161.8 mg
5. 185.3 mg

Unit 13 Clinical Calculations

Practice: Solve Using the Label Factor Method (pages 268–324)

1. 0.5 tab	41. 2 tab	81. Give 1.3 ml, Discard 0.7 ml
2. 0.5 tab	42. 3 cap	
3. 0.5 tab	43. 0.5 tab	82. 3 ml
4. 10 ml	44. 2 tab	83. 1.3 ml
5. 2 cap	45. 4 tab	84. 1.2 ml
6. 2 tab	46. 1 tab	85. 2.3 ml
7. 2 cap	47. 0.5 tab	86. 11 m
8. 3 tab	48. 10 ml	87. 0.2 ml
9. 12.5 ml	49. 0.6 ml	88. 0.8 ml
10. 2 tab	50. 1 ml	89. 0.8 ml
11. 2.5 ml	51. 1.7 ml	90. 0.2 ml
12. 6 ml	52. 0.5 ml	91. 0.3 ml
13. 13.5 or 15 ml	53. 0.8 ml	92. 1.5 ml
14. 2.5 ml	54. 1 ml	93. 1.6 ml
15. 7 ml	55. 1.2 ml	94. 1.4 ml
16. 800 mg	56. 0.75 ml	95. 0.4 ml
17. 3 tab	57. 0.6 ml	96. 1.3 ml
18. 22.5 ml	58. 2 ml	97. 1.7 ml
19. 2 tab	59. 1.5 ml	98. 0.7 ml
20. 2 tab	60. 4 m	99. 1.7 ml
21. 2.4 ml	61. 0.5 ml	100. 1 ml
22. 2 tab	62. 0.5 ml	101. 0.5 ml
23. 18 or 20 ml	63. 0.4 ml	102. 2.4 ml
24. 2 tab	64. 0.5 ml	103. 1 ml
25. 0.5 tab	65. 4 ml	104. 3 ml
26. 2 tab	66. 0.6 ml	105. 0.6 ml
27. 3 cap	67. 0.7 ml	106. 1.5 ml
28. 3 cap	68. 1.4 ml	107. 0.5 ml
29. 1 ½ tab	69. 0.7 ml	108. 0.05 ml
30. 3 tab	70. 9 m	109. 0.4 ml
31. 10 ml	71. 1.6 ml	110. 0.7 ml
32. 1 tab	72. 0.7 ml	111. 31 gtt
33. 1 tab	73. 0.5 ml	112. 31 gtt
34. 10 ml	74. 0.7 ml	113. 26 gtt
35. 2.5 ml	75. 4 ml	114. 42 gtt
36. 10 ml	76. 0.8 ml	115. 63 gtt
37. 1 tab	77. 1.5 ml	116. 31 gtt
38. 2 cap	78. 0.5 ml	117. 10 gtt
39. 0.5 tab	79. 1 or 1.1 ml	118. 36 gtt
40. 4 tab	80. 9 or 10 m	119. 21 gtt

120. 6 gtt
121. 8 gtt
122. 28 gtt
123. 21 gtt
124. 38 gtt
125. 25 gtt
126. 36 gtt
127. 14 gtt
128. 42 gtt
129. 31 gtt
130. 83 gtt
131. 25 gtt
132. 42 gtt
133. 7 gtt
134. 150 gtt
135. a. 20 ml
     b. 110 gtt
136. a. Add 30 ml
     b. 10 gtt
137. 10 hr 24 min
138. a. Add 7 ml
     b. 107 ml
139. 35 gtt
140. a. Add 21 ml
     b. 30 gtt
141. 100 gtt
142. a. Add 1.5 ml
     b. 10 gtt
143. a. Flow rate: 12 gtt
     b. 8 hr 18 min
144. 60 U
145. 30 gtt
146. a. 375 mcg/min
     b. 28 ml
     c. 28 gtt
     d. 13.4 mcg/gtt
147. a. 23.5 U/min
     b. 50 ml
     c. 50 gtt
148. a. 310.4 mcg/min
     b. 93 ml
     c. 93 gtt
     d. 3.3 mcg/gtt

149. a. 822.7 mcg/min
     b. 99 ml
     c. 99 gtt
     d. 8.3 mcg/gtt
150. a. 886 mcg/min
     b. 66 ml
     c. 66 gtt
     d. 13.4 mcg/gtt
151. a. 198.2 mcg/min
     b. 59 ml
     c. 59 gtt
     d. 3.4 mcg/gtt
152. a. 200 mcg/ml
     b. Lower: 45 mcg/min
        Upper: 135 mcg/min
     c. Lower: 14 ml/hr
        or 14 gtt/min
        Upper: 41 ml/hr
        or 41 gtt/min
     d. 3.2 mcg/gtt
     e. 60.8 mcg/min
153. 21 ml
154. a. 8 ml
     b. 27 gtt
155. 7 hr 6 min
156. a. 6 ml
     b. 106 gtt
157. a. 5.9 ml
     b. 106 gtt
158. a. 10 ml
     b. 28 gtt
159. 60 min
160. a. 150 gtt
     b. 75 gtt
161. 24,000 U
162. a. 1.5 ml
     b. 3 min
163. 70 mg
164. a. 7.5 ml
     b. 5 min
165. a. 1.1 ml
     b. 1 min 6 sec

166. a. 0.8 ml
     b. 0.32 min or 19 sec
167. 400 kcal
168. 170 kcal
169. 70 kcal
170. 165 kcal
171. 1 tab
172. 2.5 ml
173. 3 tab
174. 0.1 ml
175. 2 cap
176. 7 ml
177. 0.6 ml
178. 5 ml
179. 16.7 ml
180. 13.6 ml
181. 0.55 ml
182. a. 325 mcg/min
     b. 39 ml/hr
183. 6.2 ml
184. 0.68 ml
185. 7.7 ml
186. 32.9 mg
187. 1.9 ml
188. 0.16 mg
189. 0.07 mg
190. 0.38 mg
191. 0.65 ml
192. 16 ml

193. 0.4 ml
194. 0.6 ml
195. 15 ml
196. 0.7 ml
197. 6 ml
198. 2 ml
199. 3.1 ml
200. 0.88 ml
201. 2 ml
202. 715.8 mg/24 hr
203. 1.3 ml/dose
204. 2 ml
205. 0.8 ml
206. 1.7 ml
207. 50 Gm
208. 5 ml
209. 10 mU
210. 10 ml
211. 500 kcal
212. 32,730 μg
213. 150 ml
214. 2 cap
215. 400 mcg
216. 26 ml
217. 40 ml
218. 0.7 ml
219. 2000 mg
220. 133 gtt

Appendix A   Arithmetic Review

Roman Numerals (page 325)

A. Express as Roman Numerals.

1. VI
2. L
3. III
4. XII
5. XXIV
6. XLVI
7. XVII
8. XXXVIII
9. XXV
10. IX

B. Express as Arabic Numerals

1. 47	6. 7
2. 29	7. 2
3. 5	8. 66
4. 112	9. 309
5. 1933	10. 13

Addition (pages 325–326)
Add Whole Numbers

1. 28	6. 1090	11. 29	16. 355
2. 25	7. 1289	12. 65	17. 1169
3. 58	8. 772	13. 66	18. 9399
4. 145	9. 13,821	14. 340	19. 6249
5. 143	10. 33,407	15. 1571	20. 59,881

Subtraction (page 326)
Subtract Whole Numbers

1. 23	6. 248	11. 11	16. 6398
2. 177	7. 12,473	12. 18	17. 216
3. 4967	8. 113	13. 169	18. 473
4. 3052	9. 125	14. 262	19. 30,915
5. 32	10. 883	15. 144	20. 23,910

Multiplication (page 326)
Multiply Numbers

1. 32	6. 14,007	11. 76	16. 139,867
2. 312	7. 349,888	12. 126	17. 21,177
3. 78,372	8. 555,384	13. 408	18. 319,600
4. 135	9. 107,019	14. 1116	19. 27,696,452
5. 13,013	10. 219,900	15. 20,224	20. 986,000

Division (page 327)
Division Problems

1. 5	6. 343.3	11. 21	16. 437.7
2. 11.8	7. 11.6	12. 81	17. 1620.9
3. 20.5	8. 20.4	13. 202	18. 19.8
4. 308.3	9. 24.2	14. 231.7	19. 1840.6
5. 181.8	10. 15.5	15. 399.6	20. 184.3

Fractions (pages 327–334)

A. Reduce to Lowest Terms

1. $\dfrac{1}{3}$

2. $\dfrac{1}{3}$

3. $\dfrac{1}{2}$

4. $\dfrac{1}{5}$

5. $\dfrac{1}{11}$

6. $\dfrac{1}{4}$

7. $\dfrac{9}{10}$

8. $\dfrac{1}{4}$

9. $\dfrac{9}{40}$

10. $\dfrac{1}{6}$

B. Convert to Improper Fractions

1. $\dfrac{11}{4}$

2. $\dfrac{71}{9}$

3. $\dfrac{53}{10}$

4. $\dfrac{49}{4}$

5. $\dfrac{20}{3}$

6. $\dfrac{47}{5}$

7. $\dfrac{5}{3}$

8. $\dfrac{3}{2}$

9. $\dfrac{52}{5}$

10. $\dfrac{51}{6}$

C. Convert to Mixed Numbers (reduce to lowest terms)

1. $4\dfrac{1}{6}$

2. $6\dfrac{1}{3}$

3. $18\dfrac{4}{5}$

4. $7\dfrac{3}{4}$

5. $1\dfrac{5}{11}$

6. $3\dfrac{1}{13}$

7. $13\dfrac{5}{9}$

8. $5\dfrac{10}{23}$

9. $20\dfrac{1}{2}$

10. $49\dfrac{1}{2}$

D. Add Fractions (change to mixed numbers and reduce to lowest terms)

1. $\dfrac{11}{9} = 1\dfrac{2}{9}$

2. $\dfrac{4}{4} = 1$

3. $\dfrac{7}{6} = 1\dfrac{1}{6}$

4. $\dfrac{5}{12}$

5. $\dfrac{9}{15} = \dfrac{3}{5}$

6. $\dfrac{48}{90} = \dfrac{8}{15}$

7. $\dfrac{13}{12} = 1\dfrac{1}{12}$

8. $\dfrac{16}{10} = 1\dfrac{3}{5}$

9. $\dfrac{13}{6} = 2\dfrac{1}{6}$

10. $\dfrac{94}{48} = 1\dfrac{23}{24}$

11. $\dfrac{3}{2} = 1\dfrac{1}{2}$

12. $\dfrac{3}{3} = 1$

13. $\dfrac{7}{8}$

14. $\dfrac{21}{12} = 1\dfrac{3}{4}$

15. $\dfrac{48}{36} = 1\dfrac{1}{3}$

16. $\dfrac{19}{12} = 1\dfrac{7}{12}$

17. $\dfrac{27}{60} = \dfrac{9}{20}$

18. $\dfrac{48}{64} = \dfrac{3}{4}$

19. $\dfrac{170}{100} = 1\dfrac{7}{10}$

20. $\dfrac{141}{72} = 1\dfrac{23}{24}$

E. Subtract Fractions (change to mixed numbers and reduce to lowest terms)

1. $\dfrac{4}{6} = \dfrac{2}{3}$

2. $\dfrac{1}{7}$

3. $\dfrac{4}{14} = \dfrac{2}{7}$

4. $\dfrac{1}{4}$

5. $\dfrac{13}{36}$

6. $\dfrac{25}{33}$

7. $\dfrac{42}{10} = 4\dfrac{1}{5}$

8. $\dfrac{210}{30} = 7$

9. $\dfrac{94}{21} = 4\dfrac{10}{21}$

10. $\dfrac{170}{40} = 4\dfrac{1}{4}$

11. $\dfrac{1}{4}$

12. $\dfrac{5}{12}$

13. $\dfrac{1}{8}$

14. $\dfrac{1}{8}$

15. $\dfrac{114}{216} = \dfrac{19}{36}$

16. $\dfrac{28}{8} = 3\dfrac{1}{2}$

17. $\dfrac{70}{50} = 1\dfrac{2}{5}$

18. $\dfrac{8}{15}$

19. $\dfrac{70}{21} = 3\dfrac{1}{3}$

20. $\dfrac{38}{6} = 6\dfrac{1}{3}$

F. Multiply Fractions

1. $\dfrac{18}{35}$

2. $\dfrac{3}{20}$

3. $\dfrac{1}{5}$

4. $36\dfrac{2}{3}$

5. 16

6. 33

7. $51\dfrac{3}{7}$

8. 68

9. $21\dfrac{7}{8}$

10. $4\dfrac{47}{50}$

G. Divide Fractions

1. 2

2. $\dfrac{1}{3}$

3. $\dfrac{23}{44}$

4. 4

5. $1\dfrac{5}{8}$

6. 2

7. $1\dfrac{2}{7}$

8. $\dfrac{9}{14}$

9. $8\dfrac{2}{3}$

10. $3\dfrac{12}{37}$

Decimals (pages 337–342)

A. Write in Numbers

1. 24.2
2. 10.4
3. 16.29
4. 30.15
5. 0.261

6. 3.003
7. 0.0009
8. 32.0027
9. 0.00006
10. 25.00085

B. Change to Fractions (reduce to lowest terms)

1. $\dfrac{5}{10} = \dfrac{1}{2}$

2. $\dfrac{4}{10} = \dfrac{2}{5}$

3. $\dfrac{53}{100}$

4. $\dfrac{25}{100} = \dfrac{1}{4}$

5. $\dfrac{16}{100} = \dfrac{4}{25}$

6. $\dfrac{35}{100} = \dfrac{7}{20}$

7. $\dfrac{548}{1000} = \dfrac{137}{250}$

8. $\dfrac{973}{1000}$

9. $\dfrac{4535}{10,000} = \dfrac{907}{2000}$

10. $\dfrac{7246}{10,000} = \dfrac{3623}{5000}$

C. Change to Decimals

1. 0.3
2. 0.2
3. 0.4
4. 0.8
5. 0.8

6. 0.9
7. 0.5
8. 0.4
9. 0.3
10. 0.4

D. Add Decimals

1. 1.96
2. 30.30
3. 15.115
4. 31.095
5. 212.215

6. 174.086
7. 89.4406
8. 2536.74636
9. 36.282716
10. 247.3781

E. Subtract Decimals

1. 22.15
2. 382.092
3. 1.68
4. 89.1664
5. 172.2362

6. 0.850648
7. 16.8914
8. 10.7187
9. 768.992
10. 677.3118

F. Round off Decimals

1. 2.3
2. 3.4
3. 32.7
4. 16.79
5. 41.11

6. 15.40
7. 3.290
8. 291.635
9. 782.5
10. 2.7

G. Multiply Decimals

1. 13.04
2. 8.15
3. 299.52
4. 107.2162
5. 6003.46

6. 0.005
7. 0.0522
8. 0.223248
9. 1.638
10. 21.249

H. Divide Decimals

1. 40
2. 2.8
3. 2.9
4. 4.5
5. 8.6

6. 0.1
7. 3
8. 14.8
9. 2018.2
10. 0.1

Accountability
  label factor method, 16
  nurse, 79
Accuracy, label factor method, 16
Addition, 325–326
Administration route, 76
Answer label
  determining, 3, 4–5
  identifying, 5, 6
Apothecaries system of
    measurement, 24–29
  abbreviations, 24–25
  comparing units, 26, 27
  converting units within, 26–29
  household system of measurement
    approximate equivalents, 36
    conversion, 36–44
  metric system of measurement
    approximate equivalents, 36
    conversion, 36–44
  notation, 25–26
  units, 24–25
Arithmetic review, 325–342

Body surface area
  label factor method, 265–266
  nomogram, 263–264
  pediatric dosage, 263–264
  starting factor, 268
Body weight
  intravenous medication
    dosage, 204–210
    flow rate, 204–210
  parenteral medication, calculations
    based on, 115–118
  pediatric dosage, 248–253
  starting factor, 267
Bolus, intravenous medication, label
    factor method calculation,
    176–177
Brand name, 49
Buccal route, 45

Cannula
  intravenous medication, 163
  intravenous solution, 163
Capsule, 46
  administration, performance
    criteria, 82–83
Catheter
  intravenous medication, 163
  intravenous solution, 163
Central venous catheter, intravenous
    medication, 171–173, 174
Child
  intramuscular injection, 246, 247
  intravenous medication, 247–248,
    257–262
  intravenous solution, 247–248,
    257–262
Coated tablet, 46
Concentration factor, 210
Conversion equation
  formulating, 3, 6–13
  setting up, 12–13
  solving, 3–4, 13–15, 14–15
Conversion factor, 2, 6, 7
  constant relationship, 6
  defined, 2
  sequence, 8–9
  variable relationship, 6

Decimal, 337–342
Deltoid site, intramuscular injection,
    137
Desire over have times quantity
    method, 1
Dimensional analysis. *See* Label
    factor method
Division, 327
Documentation
  intravenous medication, 239
  intravenous solution, 239
  medication, 76–78
Dorsogluteal site, intramuscular
    injection, 136–137

Dosage calculation, 49
Dosage strength, 49
Drop factor
    infusion set, 166
    label reading, 166
Drug distribution system, 78–79
Drug infusion rate, intravenous
        medication, 196–204
Drug name, 49

Elixir, rounding off, 48–49
Enteric coated tablet, 46
Equivalent
    appoximate, 9–10
    identifying, 10

Flow rate
    infusion pump, 183–186
    intravenous medication, 182–183
        body weight, 204–210
        calculation, 189–196
        label factor method calculation,
            176–177
        specified infusion rate, 177–178,
            180–182
        specified total infusion time, 177,
            178–180
    starting factor, 268
Fraction, 327–336

Handling precautions
    needle, 138–140
    syringe, 138–140
Heparin, subcutaneous injection,
        149–150
    performance criteria, 149–150
Household system of measurement,
        30–34
    abbreviations, 31
    apothecaries system of
        measurement
        approximate equivalents, 36
        conversion, 36–44
    comparing units, 31–32
    converting units within, 32–34

metric system of measurement
    approximate equivalents, 36
    conversion, 36–44
    notation, 31, 32
    units, 30–31
Hyperalimentation, 224

Infant
    intramuscular injection, 246, 247
    intravenous medication, 247–248,
        257–262
    intravenous solution, 247–248,
        257–262
    parenteral medication, 246–248
Infusion
    intravenous medication, 163–166
    intravenous solution, 163–166
Infusion pump
    flow rate, 183–186
    intravenous medication, 183–186
Infusion rate, intravenous
        medication, label factor
        method calculation, 176–177
Infusion set, drop factor, 166
Infusion site
    intravenous medication, 236
    intravenous solution, 236
Infusion time
    intravenous medication
        calculation, 186–187
        label factor method calculation,
            176–177
    starting factor, 268
Inhalation administration, 76
Injection, 76
Insulin
    administration, 157–161
        performance criteria, 160–161
    injection, 159–160
    label reading, 153–157
    preparations, 151–153
Insulin syringe, 91, 157
Intradermal injection, 132–133
Intradermal route, 90
Intramuscular injection, 134–138
    child, 246, 247

deltoid site, 137
dorsogluteal site, 136–137
infant, 246, 247
rectus femoris site, 138, 139
vastus lateralis site, 137–138, 139
ventrogluteal site, 135–136
Z-track, 147–149
    performance criteria, 147–149
Intramuscular route, 90
Intravenous bolus, intravenous
    medication, 219–224
Intravenous medication
    adjustment, 228–233
        performance criteria, 243–244
    administration, 235–244
    assessment, performance criteria,
        243–244
    body weight
        dosage, 204–210
        flow rate, 204–210
    bolus, label factor method
        calculation, 176–177
    calculation, 162–234
    cannula, 163
    catheter, 163
    central venous catheter, 171–173,
        174
    child, 247–248, 257–262
    documentation, 239
    drug concentration, 198–204
    drug infusion rate, 196–204
    equipment, 163
    equipment handling precautions,
        238–239
    flow rate, 182–183
        body weight, 204–210
        calculation, 189–196
        label factor method calculation,
            176–177
        specified infusion rate, 177–178,
            180–182
        specified total infusion time, 177,
            178–180
    infant, 247–248, 257–262
    infusion, 163–166
    infusion pump, 183–186

infusion rate, label factor method
    calculation, 176–177
infusion site, 236
infusion time
    calculation, 186–187
    label factor method calculation,
        176–177
intermittent administration,
    170–173
intravenous bolus, 219–224
intravenous piggyback, 170, 171
intravenous regulator, 173–176
intravenous setup, performance
    criteria, 239–241
label reading, 166, 168–170
needle, 163
nursing assessment, 228–233
nursing role, 236–238
over-the-needle type catheter
    startup, performance criteria,
        241–243
saline lock, 170–171, 173
solution volume, 198–204
termination, performance criteria,
    243–244
tritrated infusion, 210–219
volume control set, 170, 172
Intravenous piggyback, intravenous
    medication, 170, 171
Intravenous regulator, intravenous
    medication, 173–176
Intravenous solution
    adding medications, 188–189,
        196–204
        flow rate, 189–196
    adjustment, 228–233
        performance criteria, 243–244
    administration, 235–244
    assessment, performance criteria,
        243–244
    calculation, 162–234
    cannula, 163
    catheter, 163
    child, 247–248, 257–262
    containers, 167
    documentation, 239

equipment, 163
equipment handling precautions,
238–239
infant, 247–248, 257–262
infusion, 163–166
infusion site, 236
intravenous setup, performance
criteria, 239–241
label reading, 166, 168–170
needle, 163
nursing assessment, 228–233
nursing role, 236–238
over-the-needle type catheter
startup, performance criteria,
241–243
termination, performance criteria,
243–244

Kardex, 76–78, 85–89

Label factor method, 1–16
accountability, 16
accuracy, 16
advantages, 2
application, 3–4, 15–16
body surface area, 265–266
clinical calculations, 267–324
defined, 2
equation solving, 13
pediatric dosage, 265–266
percentage solution, 344–346
rationale, 4–5
relationships, 4–5
steps, 2–3
Label reading, 49
drop factor, 166
insulin, 153–157
intravenous medication, 166,
168–170
intravenous solution, 166, 168–170
parenteral medication, 99–104
Liquid medication, 46
administration, performance
criteria, 83–84
administration via syringe,
performance criteria, 84–85
rounding off, 48–49

Medex, 76–78, 85–89
Medication
administration rules, 79–80
nurse, 79
recording, 76–78
Medication order, oral medication,
71, 72
Medicine cup, oral medication, 46–47
Metric system of measurement,
17–23
abbreviations, 17, 18
apothecaries system of
measurement
approximate equivalents, 36
conversion, 36–44
basic units, 17, 18
comparing units, 17–19
converting units within, 19–23
household system of measurement
approximate equivalents, 36
conversion, 36–44
notation, 17, 18
prefixes, 18
Multiple-dose vial, parenteral
medication, 98
dosage calculation, 105–115
Multiplication, 326

Needle, 92–93
handling precautions, 138–140
intravenous medication, 163
intravenous solution, 163
Nomogram, body surface area,
263–264
Normal saline solution, 30
Nurse
accountability, 79
medication, 79
Nursing assessment
intravenous medication, 228–233
intravenous solution, 228–233

Oral medication
abbreviation, 73–76
dosage, 73
preparations, 73
routes, 74

special instructions, 75
times, 74
administration, 71–89, 80–81
    performance criteria, 82–85
calculation, 45–70, 60–70
calculations based on body weight,
    57–60
defined, 45
forms, 45–46
medication order, 71, 72
medicine cup, 46–47
pediatric dosage, 245–246,
    248–253
    body weight, 248–253
rounding off, 47–49

Parenteral administration, 76
Parenteral medication
administration, 132–161, 140–141
    performance criteria, 141–146
body weight, calculations based on,
    115–118
calculation, 90–131
defined, 90
forms, 97–98
infant, 246–248
injection sites, 132–138
injection techniques, 132–138
label reading, 99–104
multiple-dose vial, 98
    dosage calculation, 105–115
pediatric dosage, 245–246
pre-filled cartridge, 98, 99
rounding off, 95
routes, 90
single-dose ampule, 97
single-dose vial, 98
    dosage calculation, 105–115
subcutaneous injection, 149
unit, 118–122
Z-track, 147–149
Parenteral nutrition, 224–228
Pediatric dosage, 245–266
body surface area, 263–264
body weight, 248–253
injection, 254–257
label factor method, 265–266

oral medication, 245–246, 248–253
    body weight, 248–253
parenteral medication, 245–246
Percentage solution, 343–348
    label factor method, 344–346
Peripheral parenteral nutrition, 224
Peripheral total parenteral nutrition,
    224
Physician's order sheet, oral
    medication, 71, 72
Powder form medication,
    reconstitution, 122–131
Pre-filled cartridge, parenteral
    medication, 98, 99

Ratio and proportion method, 1
Rectus femoris site, intramuscular
    injection, 138, 139
Roman numerals, 325
Rounding off
    elixir, 48–49
    liquid medication, 48–49
    oral medication, 47–49
    parenteral medication, 95
    solution, 48–49
    suspension, 48–49
    syringe, 96–97
    syrup, 48–49
    tablet, 47–48

Saline lock, intravenous medication,
    170–171, 173
Single-dose ampule, parenteral
    medication, 97
Single-dose vial, parenteral
    medication, 98
    dosage calculation, 105–115
Solid, equivalent units, 343–344
Solution, rounding off, 48–49
Starting factor, 1, 267
    body surface area, 268
    body weight, 267
    determining, 3, 4–5
    flow rate, 268
    identifying, 5, 6
    infusion time, 268

Subcutaneous injection, 133–134
  heparin, 149–150
    performance criteria, 149–150
  parenteral medication, 149
Subcutaneous route, 90
Sublingual route, 45
Subtraction, 326
Suspension, rounding off, 48–49
Sustained-release capsule, 46
Syringe, 91–92
  handling precautions, 138–140
  reading, 93–94
  rounding off, 96–97
Syrup, rounding off, 48–49

Tablet, 45–46
  administration, performance
    criteria, 82–83
  rounding off, 47–48
Titration factor, 210

Topical administration, 76
Total parenteral nutrition, 224
Trade name, 49
Tritrated infusion, intravenous
    medication, 210–219
Tuberculin syringe, 91, 92

Unit dose system, 78–79

Vastus lateralis site, intramuscular
    injection, 137–138, 139
Ventrogluteal site, intramuscular
    injection, 135–136
Volume control set, intravenous
    medication, 170, 172

Z-track
  intramuscular injection, 147–149
    performance criteria, 147–149
  parenteral medication, 147–149